Psychoanalysis

Colin Wright

Critical, Cultural and
Communications Press

Nottingham
2008

Orientations 1
Series Editor: Macdonald Daly

Psychoanalysis
by Colin Wright

First published in Great Britain by Critical, Cultural and Communications Press, 2008. Second edition with minor revisions, 2010.

Cover design by Andrew Dawson.

ISBN 9781905510078

Contents

Preface

Despite continuing reports to the contrary, psychoanalysis is not dead. It persists today, over a hundred years since its putative birth, though largely in a form with which its originator would not have been best pleased. In the Anglophone world at least, it exists primarily as a generalised cultural inheritance, and as a body of conceptual tools that theorists of all sorts have found it useful to pick up and use from time to time. Freud's dream of psychoanalysis as a widely accepted scientific and therapeutic practice may not have been realised, but his ideas continue to play a central role in both popular culture and critical intellectual activity.

This book focuses on psychoanalytic *theory*, rather than on clinical practice. The omission of any sustained engagement with therapeutic technique, analytical training, or indeed specific clinical case-studies, is regrettable for several reasons. Firstly, because Freud always arrived at his theoretical speculations via therapeutic interventions; secondly, because psychoanalysis has done so much to problematise the very distinction between theory and practice; and thirdly, because it reflects the comparative shunning of clinical psychoanalysis from within mainstream psychology. Nonetheless, this omission was necessary in order to maintain the brevity that a reader completely new to psychoanalysis would surely appreciate. Moreover, I would suggest that the decline in the popularity of *clinical* psychoanalysis is substantially off-set by the enthusiastic recent uptake of psychoanalytic *theory* in disciplines like continental philosophy, cultural studies, and political theory.[1]

My simple hope is that readers will come away from this book with both a sense of the rich breadth of the psychoanalytic movement as whole, and a firm grasp of several key concepts used in today's theoretical discourses in the humanities and beyond. Yet, their appetite whetted, I hope readers will also go on to consider the therapeutic aspect of psychoanalysis explored in more comprehensive works than this, for without an understanding of the clinical process, the theory arguably remains *only* academic. One of the primary claims of psychoanalysis is that it *does* something, that it actively intervenes, and is therefore far from being a static 'knowledge'.

The book is structured in two halves. The first deals with Freud's seminal ideas on the unconscious, repression, sexuality and culture, and therefore introduces the foundations of a Freudian 'orthodoxy'. The second effectively has two sections, with chapters 6, 7 and 8 introducing the key post-Freudian thinkers Carl Jung, Melanie Klein and Jacques Lacan.

[1] The name of Slavoj Žižek increasingly evokes this enthusiasm. He is a Professor of Sociology at Lubjiana University in Slovenia whose prodigious output since the late 1980s has pioneered a Lacanian approach to popular culture which has been very influential on film theory.

Chapters 9 and 10 address some of the important critiques of psychoanalysis coming from feminists, neuroscientists and philosophers. The second half therefore challenges the orthodoxy set up in the first. While many other post-Freudians could have been chosen for chapters 6, 7 and 8, it was felt that the very diversity of the theoretical systems of Jung, Klein and Lacan simultaneously indicated the eclecticism within the psychoanalytic movement as a whole. Crucially, the distance between Jungian 'archetypes', Kleinian 'positions', and the Lacanian 'signifier' militate against that monolithic version of psychoanalysis still occasionally built specifically for the purpose of being knocked down again. The last two chapters are intended to testify to the controversy which psychoanalysis has always inspired, and to ensure that the overall account given is balanced – even if my general aim is to advocate the relevance of psychoanalytic theory for numerous contemporary social, cultural, political and aesthetic phenomena. At the very end of the book, I have included a short supplementary bibliography designed to guide further reading.

1 What is Psychoanalysis?

The word 'psychoanalysis' conjures up various associations: the name 'Sigmund Freud'; dreams and neuroses; lying on a couch and discussing your relationship to your mother; and the idea that, when you really analyse human behaviour, it all somehow boils down to sex! However, such banal associations hardly amount to a *definition* of psychoanalysis. To give that, something much more rigorous is required. In the particular case of psychoanalysis, however, this is a very difficult task.

We can account for this difficulty in various ways. Firstly, psychoanalysis is now well over one hundred years old (there is some disagreement, but the year 1895 is generally accepted as an agreed birth-date). As a body of thought, it has developed in multiple and perhaps contradictory directions since its founding statements in the late nineteenth century. When we use the word 'psychoanalysis' then, we can be talking about any part of this complex history. Secondly, from the very beginning, psychoanalysis has been internally contested. Even Freud's own theory, while remarkably consistent in its central concerns, nonetheless shifts its paradigms and terminology many times: the early Freud is not the same as the middle or late Freud. Moreover, during Freud's own lifetime, there were numerous psychoanalysts, such as Carl Jung and Alfred Adler, who came to disagree with certain crucial tenets of 'Freudianism'. These apostates went on to formulate their own theories, so that very different interpretations of psychoanalysis were already proliferating well before Freud's death in 1939. Thirdly, this fragmentation was compounded by the various national and international associations and societies of psychoanalysis which tended to present their specific interpretations as the 'true' psychoanalysis. Because of this institutionalisation of competing orthodoxies, trying to define what psychoanalysis is has become something of a political minefield. Fourthly, in its wide-ranging travels, psychoanalysis has been taken on in different ways by different national cultures: the kind of psychoanalysis predominant in France is very different from that which exists in Britain, which is different again from the American model, and so on around the globe.

However, it is important to emphasise a fifth point that side-steps the problem of the various filters through which any definition of psychoanalysis must pass, by stressing not what psychoanalysis is, but the uses to which it has been put. We can explore four such uses.

1. As a therapy
2. As an attempted science of the mind
3. As a social theory
4. As a way of reading

Psychoanalysis as a Therapy

Freud was a doctor, and his primary hope for psychoanalysis was always that it would constitute a form of therapy. As a therapy, psychoanalysis postulates an unconscious realm of the psyche that has a profound bearing on an individual's emotional life and everyday behaviour, despite remaining outside their awareness. Such unconscious forces can create symptoms of depression, anxiety, and odd behaviour such as obsessive compulsive rituals, hysterical outbursts, or repeated negative patterns in personal relationships. Because the cause of these symptoms is unconscious, the individuals themselves cannot explain them. The role of the psychoanalyst, then, is to help the patient to bring these unconscious thoughts into consciousness, in order to understand what is causing them to feel and act in such strange ways.

In its therapeutic role, psychoanalysis is often referred to as the 'talking cure' because this process of making unconscious forces conscious is traditionally done via 'free association'. Free association simply involves the patient giving unrestrained expression to any words, thoughts, or images which leap to mind whilst on the therapist's couch. Gradually, these spontaneous associations reveal connections or complexes that can give the analyst clues as to what might be going on in the patient's unconscious. However, the most important (and difficult) moment in therapy occurs when the patient encounters a block in their ability to proceed with these free associations. This moment of 'resistance' is when the analysis has come upon the hard kernel of the unconscious forces affecting the patient's well-being. The analyst then pursues the *origins* of these unconscious forces into the patient's personal life history, where there is usually some traumatic childhood experience that has been repressed and thereby excluded from conscious recollection. The patient's resistance to analysis is born of their reluctance to face and re-experience this repressed memory, which is nonetheless struggling for some kind of expression (and finding it, in a distorted form, in their neurotic symptoms). Yet by bringing these deeply submerged experiences to intellectual and emotional awareness, it is claimed that psychoanalytic therapy can enable patients to understand the unconscious motivations behind their behaviour, and therefore to find ways of adapting that behaviour.

Although convinced of its specific value, Freud did not make any exorbitant claims for psychoanalysis as a form of therapy. For example, he remained adamant throughout his career that schizophrenia – what he called 'dementia praecox' – was not suitable for psychoanalytic forms of treatment, since sufferers were incapable of 'transference'. Transference is the process whereby a patient projects feelings associated with important figures from their previous life history, such as parents or siblings, onto the analyst. At the beginning of his own psychiatric practice, Freud viewed transference as a problem, since patients would often become aggressive towards him and withdraw from the analysis altogether. Later, he understood that this was an essential part of 'working through' their unconscious problems and the only way of breaking down their resistances. However, individuals with what he called 'narcissistic neuroses', which is to say those who were incapable of identifying with other people, were beyond the reach of psychoanalytic treatment. Freudian *therapy* therefore made few in-roads into what we might now refer to as full-blown 'mental illness' (although psychoanalytic *theory* has certainly been an important tool in describing the mechanisms of mental illness). Instead, it generally restricted itself to non-psychotic psychiatric complaints whose symptoms we are still familiar with today, such as compulsive self-harm, obsessive cleanliness, agoraphobia, melancholia and depression.

If Freud did not present psychoanalytic therapy as a panacea for all mental suffering, this is perhaps because its aim is actually comparatively modest. Psychoanalysis does not promise cure in any final sense, but aspires instead to the attainment of a level of normality and integration acceptable to the culture and society in which the patient lives. After all, a traumatic event in someone's past does not cease to exert its effects just because it has been recalled and faced. Nonetheless, psychoanalytic therapy does claim to be able to resolve the psychological problems caused by the repression of this experience or feeling, which were in turn preventing that individual from enjoying a full and normal social life. In this sense, psychoanalysis deals with constructions of social norms, and the emotional price which is paid for deviance from those norms: its therapeutic goal is therefore to rectify stalled or defective processes of socialisation. This can be seen as a conservative side of psychoanalysis, in that it reinforces the status quo. On the other hand, however, there is a much more critical aspect implicit in psychoanalytic therapy which emphasises the repressive nature of these social norms themselves. Such a view opens up the possibility of blaming society for the neuroses it creates, rather than individuals for suffering from them, and this can be seen as the radical or critical side of psychoanalysis.

In general then, the twentieth century, with its rampant modernity, traumatic world wars, ethnic cleansing, and threat of nuclear annihilation, proved fertile ground for psychoanalysis as a therapy. After World War II, psychoanalysis was the dominant force in psychology, and remains the foundation of all dynamic approaches to psychotherapy today, particularly in cognitive psychology and attachment theory, as well as family and group therapies.

Psychoanalysis as an Attempted Science

Throughout his writings, Freud is concerned with the scientific status of psychoanalysis. In this, he is very much a product of his time. The nineteenth century – which witnessed, in the industrial revolution, the unleashing of technological modernity, and, in Darwinism, the apparent victory of rational observation over theological doctrine – was a century obsessed with science. This was particularly true of Vienna, Freud's home town in Austria, and one of the most culturally and intellectually vibrant cities in Europe. Freud's general intellectual milieu, then, as well as the radical nature of what he was proposing, demanded that a claim to scientific status be made on behalf of psychoanalysis. But Freud's professional training too, as a medical doctor with a particular interest in physiology (his first piece of research was into the anatomy of the eel!), also led him to present psychoanalysis as, at least potentially, a scientific form of knowledge. Thus, in describing the structures and tendencies within the human psyche, he repeatedly makes references to biological and even chemical processes. He also generally tries to ground his theoretical speculations in the observation of neurotic patients, treating the psychoanalyst's office rather like a laboratory. Although psychoanalysis has certainly taken on a theoretical life of its own since Freud, it still retains roots in clinical practice and therefore in lived experience. Just as Darwin based his theory of natural selection on observations of the natural world, so psychoanalysis bases its theory of the unconscious on observations of the psychic world of human beings.

However, whether psychoanalysis can in fact be described as a science is still very much open to debate. There have been out-and-out critics, like Hans Eysenck,[1] who dismisses psychoanalysis precisely because it is not scientific enough. There have even been psychoanalysts, like H. J. Home,[2] who themselves deny that psychoanalysis is, or should try to be, a science. There have also been hybrid arguments, like that of Charles Rycroft,[3] who claims that psychoanalysis creates a bridge between the biological sciences and the humanities. But in the 1950s, fully halfway into the life of the discipline, Jacques Lacan was still admitting that psychoanalysis was not yet a science.[4] All of these arguments, of course, depend on what notion of science is being assumed. If science is understood along classical Newtonian lines, as a practice that must be measurable, conducted in controlled conditions, and capable of verification by repetition, then

[1] Eysenck, H. J. *Fact and Fiction in Psychology* (Harmondsworth: Penguin, 1965).
[2] Home, H. J. 'The Concept of the Mind', *International Journal of Psycho-Analysis* 47 (1966), pp. 43-9.
[3] Rycroft, Charles. *Psychoanalysis and Beyond* (London: Hogarth Press, 1991).
[4] Lacan, Jacques. *Écrits*, trans. Bruce Fink (London: Norton, 2006).

psychoanalysis obviously falls very far short of being scientific. Human emotions are not conducive to quantitative analysis. Human beings generally live very complex lives, so that isolating variables is almost impossible. And finally, because psychoanalytic therapy constitutes a dynamic intervention into the object of its own study, it follows that, far from verifying psychoanalytic hypotheses, simple repetition might be said to contradict those hypotheses.

And yet, a more generous understanding of science, as simply the accumulation of systematic knowledge based on empirical observation, allows psychoanalysis to make a much more plausible claim to scientific status. After all, Freud and his successors have undoubtedly created a systematic and yet flexible vocabulary for describing observable tendencies in human behaviour. They have also constructed explanatory models that seem to have genuine descriptive, even predictive, power when applied to actual living people. That is, psychoanalysis continues to be practised because it seems to continue to describe the way people behave and feel. Moreover, because of its therapeutic dimension, psychoanalysis is arguably more concerned with tangible results than with absolute logical coherence. Indeed, one could argue that the attempt to prove the scientific worth of psychoanalysis may have been a response to nineteenth century rationalism, and, moreover, that this should be seen in the context of the torrid objections to which psychoanalysis was initially subjected.

In fact, this debate can be subsumed under the broader debate about the scientific status of psychology generally, as an attempted science of the mind, as psychoanalysis can be seen as that branch of psychology which advocates the existence of an unconscious.

Psychoanalysis as a Social Theory

As already stated, psychoanalysis deals with what is considered normal and abnormal, so that it also deals with society at large, as the place where these values are constructed and circulated. It is society – through individuals like policeman and judges, and institutions like schools and workplaces – that determines what counts as normal, as well as what disciplinary measures result from flouting that 'normality'. Neurotics usually seek psychoanalytic therapy because they are only too aware that their behaviour is seen by the wider world as weird, irrational, embarrassing, or even crazy. However, what is judged weird, irrational, embarrassing, and even crazy is partially dependent upon the society in which the individuals live, as well as their place within it. One way to think of this is in terms of cultural differences around displays of grief: while tremendous wailing and gesticulating and even writhing around on the floor might appear excessive to a restrained British person, to a resident of a Middle Eastern country, it might register as quite normal. Conversely, grim, tight-lipped stoicism in the wake of the loss of a loved one might appear totally pathological to a Middle Eastern person. Clearly, in such different social and cultural contexts, neurotic symptoms will arise in different ways and for different reasons. One should probably add to these influential differences the factors of race, class and gender (particularly because classical psychoanalysis seems largely blind to its own roots in the social and cultural norms of the European male bourgeoisie).

Nonetheless, in so far as psychoanalysis describes the formation of subjectivity from infancy, through adolescence, and on into adulthood, it also describes the individual's progressive encounters with various agents of these societal norms. This process obviously starts with parents (especially the father), but soon moves on to teachers and school peers, bosses at work, even traffic wardens, tax collectors, and perhaps university lecturers. These figures have in common a certain insistence on rules and regulations and 'good' behaviour, as well as, usually, the capacity to exert institutionally recognised punishments for 'bad' behaviour. Part of 'growing up' then, is submission to wider social norms and acknowledgment of the violence with which those norms are backed up. The primary insight of psychoanalysis as a social theory is therefore that society is fundamentally based on the repression of instinctual drives, and that this repression is reinforced by law, broadly conceived.

According to this view, society, as an ordered, usually hierarchical and rational place, begins with the renunciation of total freedom. We cannot just go around doing whatever we want whenever we feel like it, as that would result in utter chaos. Rather, we must defer our immediate desires in the interests of a wider collective goal. Think of animals that hunt in packs as a very basic social unit. The assignment of roles in such a pack – shepherding prey into a collectively organised trap, as opposed to directly catching and killing that prey – demands the renunciation of immediate gratification, on the understanding that some form of gratification will be met with later on. Hunting in packs is predicated upon the deferment of pleasure. In an intuitive sense then, co-operation involves giving up total selfishness. In fact, this was the theory of the seminal political philosopher, Thomas Hobbes. In his book *Leviathan* (1651), Hobbes claimed that, left to their own devices, people live in a cruel state of nature in which everybody is relentlessly selfish and life is 'solitary, poor, nasty, brutish and short'. The only way out of this state is to submit to a single, all-powerful sovereign who can enforce law and order. For Hobbes, who was writing just after the tumult of the English Civil War, this was an eloquent argument for a society based on centralised, even personalised, power, and the renunciation of certain freedoms in the interests of social stability.

Freud would agree with Hobbes that society involves controlling our primordial instincts. However, according to psychoanalysis, even in a society governed by an all-powerful sovereign, the aggressive and destructive instincts that characterise the state of nature do not simply evaporate after the imagined signing of this social contract. On the contrary, they remain and have to be actively repressed, which is to say, socialised. For full socialisation to take place (although it is an on-going process, rather than a single event), the psychoanalytic social theorist would argue that there needs to be a combination of three key components. Firstly, a prohibitive law; secondly, an identification with the agent of that law; and thirdly, an internalisation of that agent, so that the individual becomes self-policing. Clearly, society would be impossible to regulate if people were only law-abiding when they happened to be within the eye-line of a policeman! Much more efficient is the setting up of an *internal* policeman, which Freud, in his later career, was to refer to as the 'super-ego'.

It should be obvious that all of this is more complicated than simply saying that as people get older they encounter various external forces which domesticate them into being good citizens, rather as toddlers get potty-trained. For according to psychoanalysis, subjectivity itself emerges from such encounters and cannot be separated from them. In a very subtle way – and this is what has been so problematic for attempts to reconcile Freud with emancipatory politics – the subject that is formed by these encounters ends up investing in, and identifying with, the very social forces which repress it. On this view, the relationship between the dominators and the dominated becomes analogous to the complicity between sadists (people who get pleasure from other people's pain) and masochists (people who get pleasure from having pain inflicted on them). Just as masochists willingly expose themselves to sadistic treatment, so social subjects are magnetically attracted to the forces that socialise them. For some radical social theorists influenced by psychoanalysis who were writing just after World War II, this complicity between subjection and subjectivity was the only way to understand the participation of the German people in Hitler's Final Solution. By the time of the sexual revolution of the 1960s, many of these same theorists were arguing that the solution to this sado-masochistic structure of power lay in overthrowing the social order that demanded such severe repression in the first place. On this point, Freud was perhaps more ambivalent, arguing that civilization is composed of an unceasing play between destructive *and* affirmative forces. Nonetheless, he was certainly critical of the hypocrisy of the prim Victorian moral order that surrounded him – even though it was that order which provided him with so many neurotics to treat and study!

Psychoanalysis as a Way of Reading

Perhaps the most unexpected way in which psychoanalysis has been taken up, at least from the point of view of Freud's aspirations for the discipline, has been as a tool within literary theory. This fact may seem rather strange, given all that we have said so far. And yet, if we set aside its larger therapeutic, scientific, and perhaps social goals, it can be seen that, in terms of its methodology, psychoanalysis was always in essence a subtle theory of reading.

After all, the classic formulations of the nature of the unconscious, which provide the very cornerstone of psychoanalysis, arose in direct conjunction with the minute analysis of *latent meanings*. Latent meanings are those that are hidden from view, but exist nonetheless. That is to say, intimations of the existence of the unconscious, elusive by its very nature, can be had only by means of the detailed interpretation of hidden meanings. Freud first 'discovered' the unconscious whilst studying two seemingly unrelated phenomena: *lapsus linguae*, or slips of the tongue ('Freudian slips'), and people's accounts of their own dreams. Both of these phenomena provided 'texts', taken in the broadest sense,. which then became the raw material for psychoanalytic analysis.

Yet these texts, rather like literary texts, are not at all straightforward. What you see (or read) of the unconscious is not what you get. We can all confirm this if we think of our own dreams, which often strike us as utterly bizarre. This is because the unconscious occupies a realm somehow outside, or before, or below, literal language. Freud said again and again that the unconscious knows nothing of time, or space, or causality. The unconscious ignores the rules which govern rational experience, so that any messages which float up from its mysterious depths are unlikely to be readily legible to the average mind trained (again by socialising processes) in rational forms of interpretation. It does not follow, however, that such messages are meaningless or irrational. Indeed, a large portion of Freud's early work consisted in demonstrating the symbolic grammar of unconscious utterances, and therefore in providing a theoretical system for interpreting, for consciousness, the enigmatic texts of the *un*conscious, such as slips of the tongue, dreams, and of course neurotic symptoms.

The major work which underpins the literary theoretical appropriation of psychoanalysis is Freud's monumental *The Interpretation of Dreams* (1900). It is here that, through painstaking readings of a host of collated dreams, Freud makes the distinction between latent and manifest meanings, and between the primary processes of the unconscious and the secondary processes of consciousness. It is also where he manages to identify the four mechanisms of what he calls the dream-work, but which apply to all primary or unconscious processes (and are therefore at work in neurotic symptoms as well): they are 'condensation', 'displacement', 'symbolisation', and 'contradiction'. Condensation involves at least two mental images or meanings being combined in a single mental image which is nonetheless invested with meaning from both of its composite elements. Displacement is the process whereby psychic energy, which Freud calls 'cathexis', can be transmitted from one mental image to another. Symbolism refers to the capacity of something to stand for something else, the stereotypical example in terms of unconscious symbolism being, say, an umbrella, or a pen, or even a car, standing in for the penis. Finally, the unconscious displays a remarkable tolerance for contradiction, so that during dreams the most absurd and indeed impossible situations are experienced as quite normal.

To the extent that dream-interpretation starts with the manifest content of the dream and undoes the mechanisms of the dream-work to reveal a latent (unconscious) meaning, it is a process analogous to the literary critic's interpretation of a difficult poem to arrive at its deeper signification. A psychoanalytic interpretation of a literary text can therefore settle for profiling an author's psychological make up via his or her literary works; or it can identify psychoanalytic 'themes' on the surface of a work, for example, by interpreting Shakespeare's *Hamlet* through the Oedipus complex; or it can be more radical, by applying a 'symptomatic reading' which pays attention to the gaps, silences and outright contradictions which reveal a text's 'unconscious' concerns irrespective of what its author's intentions in producing it may or may not have been.

Freud himself often utilised examples from literature, art, and ancient Greek mythology in order to explain his theories, but, through the concept of sublimation, he also sketched a psychoanalytic role for literature specifically, and culture generally. Sublimation describes the redirection of libidinal energy away from sexual aims, and towards socially validated forms of practice. Thus what we might describe as 'high culture', from the arts to the sciences, is a result of the mobilisation of psychic energy for social, rather than sexual, ends. Unlike classical Marxism, which makes such high culture a secondary superstructure built upon a material base, classical psychoanalysis really makes cultural expression a prerequisite of social life. Literature and the arts in general therefore become privileged points of entry into the inner psychological workings of social systems.

Conclusion

These are just four uses to which psychoanalysis has been put. There are many more. For instance, we could mention the use of psychoanalysis in advertising and marketing, in art, in politics, and even in warfare. Indeed, psychoanalysis is really best described as an extremely broad cultural phenomenon that has impacted on many areas of our contemporary lives, from the language we use to the films we watch. It is difficult to define precisely because, in a sense, we always already enjoy its rich legacy. But despite our initial reluctance to establish a definition of psychoanalysis, we are not absolved from looking closely at its basic claims, its pre-eminent spokespersons, and the differences between them. In what follows, we shall be looking primarily at psychoanalytical theory, with Freud, and after Freud. That is, we shall be trying to clarify the most essential ideas of the psychoanalytic approach and asking whether it still has a place in today's world, so radically different from Freud's.

2 Freud: the Unconscious

The 'discovery' of the unconscious deserves to be considered among the most profound discoveries in Western history. Its intellectual, cultural and philosophical ramifications have arguably been on a par with the seismic shocks of the Copernican Revolution, when our own planet ceased to be the centre of the known universe, and of Darwinian Evolutionism, when man became, not the elevated reflection of God's divinity, but an animal like any other. This may sound excessively grand, but, like those discoveries, the revelation of an unconscious dimension within mental life shook to the very core a powerful and widespread assumption: that of the *sovereignty of the subject*. If sovereignty is understood as the dominion of a controlling power, one can sketch with these intellectual signposts a trajectory of diminishing power: Copernicus displaced us from the centre of the universe, but at least we had dominion over our own planet ... until Darwin came along and mocked our self-importance by placing us on the same plane as the apes ... and then Freud arrived, claiming that we were not even sovereign within our own minds! This was, and remains, both shocking and challenging because it was upon the supposedly serene rationality of this sovereign subject that the 'Big Ideas' of Western thought had been hitherto based. The unconscious therefore rendered problematic everything from politics to ethics, and struck many as irrational and quite possibly immoral.

So what is the unconscious?

Parapraxes

Whenever Freud was trying to communicate his ideas about the unconscious to ordinary 'lay' people, he invariably started with 'parapraxes'. Parapraxes are simple everyday actions that are nonetheless carried out *unsuccessfully* for no obvious external reason. They are not the same as simple mistakes, however. Freud's central claim is that the lack of success characteristic of parapraxes finds its source in the existence of two opposing intentions, as if the mind were trying to do two contradictory things at once. Before we go on to look at this thesis, it should be stated that all of us are very familiar with the phenomenon of parapraxis. It is at work in the following everyday scenarios:

- Our minds suddenly go blank whilst trying to recall the name of someone we know very well.
- We repeatedly 'forget' about our appointment at the dentist.
- We consistently lose the keys to the car we should be lending to a friend.

- We blurt out 'no' even when the polite answer, and the one we *meant* to say, was 'yes'.

For Freud, such incidents are interesting for several reasons. Firstly, his analysis of them indicates the existence of the unconscious in a way that everyone can empathise with, because everybody has experienced a parapraxis. Secondly, they help to suggest that *everyone* has an unconscious, that it is a normal and essential part of psychic life that doesn't only effect neurotics (Freud's most sustained treatment of the topic comes in a book revealingly entitled *The Psychopathology of Everyday Life*). Thirdly however, the phenomenon of parapraxes also gets to the heart of why the notion of the unconscious specifically – and hence of psychoanalysis generally – often meets with such profound resistance. After all, being told that you made a mistake because at some level you intended to flies in the face of how we think of ourselves. We are accustomed to viewing ourselves as intentional beings with willpower and the capacity to direct that willpower toward goals of our own choosing. We naturally want to be completely in charge of our own actions and to undertake those actions on the basis of rational decisions. Yet according to Freud, such ultra-rational intentionality is ultimately illusory, notwithstanding our instinctive reluctance to accept this fact. This is one of the cleverest and most infuriating aspects of psychoanalysis: vehemently disagreeing with it can be interpreted as 'resistance', and thus as evidence of the very thing that is being denied!

So let us follow Freud's example then, and use parapraxes to introduce the notion of the unconscious. In fact, Freud's analysis of one kind of parapraxis has become so famous that his name is attached to it in everyday speech: the so-called 'Freudian Slip'. Because of the subtle linguistic nature of slips of the tongue, many of the examples given by Freud require fairly tortuous explications of the German language in which he wrote. However, we can start with the following example. It contains the basic ingredients of parapraxis without demanding a German dictionary:

> A president of the Lower House of our Parliament once opened the sitting with the words: 'Gentlemen, I take notice that a full quorum of members is present and I herewith declare the sitting *closed*'.[1]

This parapraxis is easily understandable, since it has a direct sense: the word 'closed' illustrates the speaker's wish to avoid this particular parliamentary session before it has even started, perhaps because it is going to be particularly uncomfortable for him personally. It is a parapraxis

[1] Freud, Sigmund. *Introductory Lectures in Psychoanalysis*, trans. James Strachey (London: Penguin, 1991), pp. 59-60.

because protocol demands that he does not express his personal wish in this way, but simply opens proceedings. So even though the speaker is speaking quite plainly, his statement contradicts what convention and the context lead one to expect. In a sense, this immediately suggests the presence of repression (he says what he is *not meant* to say). But does it necessarily indicate the existence of an unconscious, if we think of the unconscious as being antithetical to conscious awareness? Not really, as we can imagine that in this formal context the speaker may have been perfectly aware that he did not want to go through with this parliamentary session. His mistake lay in temporarily breaching this formality by allowing his own *conscious* wish to show itself in public.

In fact, Freud argues that this kind of slip of the tongue, in which an opposing intention is explicitly expressed, is comparatively rare. Most parapraxes do not have a sense that is obvious either to the listener or indeed to the speaker. Crucially, though, they do have a sense when subjected to analysis. Here, we must invoke one of Freud's German examples:

> [A] gentlemen addressed a lady in the street in the following words: 'If you will permit me, madam, I should like to *begleit-digen* you'.[2]

Freud suggests that this word, which does not exist in the German language, is a composite of two other words which do: *begleiten*, to accompany, and *beleidigen*, to insult. Here we might speculate that, like the parliamentary speaker above, this young man is experiencing a conflict between his own private wishes and the demands of public etiquette. The difference here is that the conflict does not announce itself literally, but causes a linguistic distortion that betrays and yet also disguises the contradiction: the lady in question would be hard put to realise that the gentlemen ardently hoped to get a chance to 'insult' her. Freud therefore contends that 'these obscurer cases of slips of the tongue can be explained by a convergence, a mutual "*interference*", between two different intended speeches'.[3] Again, this does not seem a radical proposal. After all, if most of us were being honest, we would admit that very often, the things we say publicly do not correspond to how we feel privately.

However, Freud's more startling claim is that we are quite unaware of one of these two contradictory intentions. Specifically, we are unaware of the disturbing intention that interfered with and distorted the disturbed intention, or the intention that we were conscious of 'meaning'. The gentleman in the example above would probably vigorously deny that he wished to 'insult' the lady at all, as this was the disturbing intention that disturbed his more laudable intention to simply accompany her. For Freud,

[2] Freud, *Introductory Lectures*, p. 58.
[3] Freud, *Introductory Lectures*, pp. 68-9.

denial does not by any means indicate that the secondary or disturbing intention does not exist (indeed, in the concept of 'resistance', it confirms its existence). What it does indicate is that the disturbing intention comes from a part of the mind that is not accessible to awareness. In other words, it originates in the unconscious.

From the moment we accept this thesis, human subjects are not fully in control of their own speech or action. Indeed, the person who makes the slip of the tongue is often the person least likely to know what it means. Only someone else, a psychoanalyst for example, can uncover the unconscious influence that is distorting the statement by putting it in its fuller context. For example, analysis may show that a person who consistently forgets the name of someone who is otherwise quite familiar to them, may unconsciously hold something against that person, and prefer not to think of them.[4] Or someone who repeatedly forgets the married name of her best friend may unconsciously disapprove of the marriage itself.[5] Or again, someone who keeps losing a significant object may harbour in their unconscious a grudge against the person who gave it to them, or, more prosaically, they may simply want to be rid of the object in a way which will not trouble their own conscience.[6] It should be obvious from these examples that the parapraxis in itself does not usually carry sufficient information to reveal the disturbing unconscious influence. On the contrary, extensive discussion may be required to lay bare the relevant circumstantial evidence. This is also the rationale behind the 'talking cure' of psychoanalytic therapy in which it is not parapraxes, but neuroses, that are considered. Freud's point is that both have their origins in the unconscious.

In fact, in speaking of the unconscious, it is practically impossible to leave aside the phenomenon of repression, since the one presupposes the other. Parapraxes illustrate this well, for can we imagine any of the preceding examples of slips of the tongue without the need to suppress an intention? It is the requirement to observe formal protocols, or rules of etiquette between the sexes, or propriety between friends and family, that makes the disturbing intention something to be censored, thereby creating the psychic (and social) conditions for it to *become* disturbing in the fullest sense. Freud noted, however, that the slip of the tongue that results from these two contradictory intentional forces never satisfies either, but is rather a *compromise* between the two: 'they constitute a half-success and a half-failure for each of the two intentions; the intention which is being challenged is neither completely suppressed nor [...] carried through quite unscathed'.[7] In the therapeutic context, Freud would go on to speak of 'compromise-formations', which, like slips of the tongue, are mental

[4] Freud, *Introductory Lectures*, p. 79.
[5] Freud, *Introductory Lectures*, p. 80.
[6] Freud, *Introductory Lectures*, p. 82.
[7] Freud, *Introductory Lectures*, p. 94.

phenomena resulting from a conflict between two psychic forces, in which both forces are partially expressed but in which, by the same token, neither are fully expressed. So a neurotic symptom and a parapraxis is a compromise between the repressed unconscious impulse, and the repressing agency of the ego.

The Nature of the Unconscious

Having at least suggested the existence of the unconscious, we must leave parapraxes behind in order to say more about the specific nature of the unconscious. This is important because we have so far been using the word in a rather limited and even misleading sense, by simplistically contrasting it to consciousness understood as subjective awareness. In fact, things are much more complicated than that.

The example of memory immediately illustrates why this should be the case. We all have a profusion of memories, but they are rarely at the forefront of our awareness. Even during the process of recollection, when certain memories do advance to the foreground of our minds, they are usually few in number, having been selected from the great mass of our total memories. Indeed, to imagine *all* of our memories simultaneously occupying our awareness would be to imagine madness! Does it follow that such memories are stored in the unconscious and, like a book from a library, are only removed for inspection when required by consciousness? In its suggestion of an easy transaction between consciousness and the unconscious, this would contradict what has already been indicated by Freud's analysis of parapraxes. That analysis demonstrated an active antagonism between the disturbing and the disturbed intentions, and suggested that this antagonism takes the form of a repression which makes the disturbing intention *inaccessible* to consciousness. In other words, while memories may not be part of our awareness at any given time, they are always available to awareness. In contrast, unconscious contents are *actively excluded from consciousness* and are only brought to its attention with great difficulty.

The word 'unconscious' therefore threatens to invoke two incompatible meanings. Firstly, 'unconscious' could mean latent, in the sense of temporarily excluded from awareness but ever available to it (as in our example of memories). Secondly, and in keeping with the fundamental claims of psychoanalysis, 'unconscious' could refer to an entirely different order of mental life that observes different psychic mechanisms altogether. Unfortunately perhaps, psychoanalysis asserts that this ambiguity cannot be cleared up by inventing two different terms for these descriptive and systematic uses of the word 'unconscious'. This is because, as already stated, repression and the unconscious are deeply inter-linked, and also because we have absolutely no access to the unconscious that is not mediated by conscious processes.

However, Freud does try to clarify this confusing situation by adopting three different but overlapping ways of approaching the unconscious. They are:

1. The Dynamic Approach
2. The Topographical Approach
3. The Economic Approach

The highest aspiration that psychoanalysis can have, according to Freud, is the synthesis of these three perspectives on the unconscious in what he called a 'metapsychological' presentation.

1. The dynamic approach simply refers to the fact that psychoanalysis does not view the unconscious as a static, unchanging entity. Such a view would apply for a theory of consciousness like that of the philosopher Immanuel Kant, which stresses the 'faculties' as fixed categories that determine all subjective experience. In contrast, psychoanalysis pictures the unconscious as a highly fluid set of processes, instincts and mechanisms that develop over time. The unconscious isn't like an underground cave that, once discovered, remains unaltered. On the contrary, it is doubly characterised by restless change on the one hand, and recognisable stages of development on the other. Freud therefore makes both 'ontogenic' and 'phylogenic' claims for the unconscious, which is to say he makes claims that operate at the level of the development of both the individual (ontogenic) and the species (phylogenic). Ontogenic arguments might apply to the specific development of sexuality in the course of an individual's personal history. Phylogenic arguments might apply to the continuities and discontinuities surrounding certain practices, such as totemism, between pre-modern and modern societies. Both assume that the unconscious is dynamic both for individuals and across historical time.

2. The topographic approach to the unconscious is one that conceives it as occupying a clearly differentiated region whose relation to the other agencies within the psyche is represented spatially (*topos* in Greek means place or space). We must be cautious here, however. Freud is very clear that this topographic view is nothing more than a useful heuristic device. He is *not* making any physiological claims pertaining to the neurological functioning of different regions of the brain (although he occasionally makes guesses in this direction). The safest way to think of the topographical approach then, is as a diagram illustrating the psychoanalytic theory of the psychic apparatus. The Freud of *The Interpretation of Dreams* builds up a topographic model of the psyche by using the terms 'unconscious', 'preconscious', 'conscious', and 'perception', representing these respectively as *Ucs.*, *Pcs.*, *Cs.* and *Pcpt.*. This system views the

unconscious as the deepest region which, as it were, presses up into the preconscious, which in turn acts as a kind of protective buffer zone between the unconscious and the uppermost layer of consciousness. It is the preconscious that censors material from the unconscious. After his discovery of a secondary form of narcissism[8] and of the death drive,[9] Freud both clarified and complicated this linear model by introducing the terms 'id', 'ego' and 'superego'. The relationship between these psychic agencies is complex, and we shall defer them until we come to consider repression.

3. In fact, it is impossible to talk about the topographic approach without reference to the economic approach, since the former is really a graphic representation of the latter. Indeed, the economic conception of psychic activity is already implicit in the dynamic approach. For if the unconscious exerts a disturbing pressure on conscious intention, as our examination of parapraxes suggested, and if analysis can reverse the distortion through which this disturbance manifests itself, it follows that unconscious forces follow a certain logic. The economic approach can therefore be thought of as theorising the regulatory logic of psychic dynamics. As the name suggests, it is essentially concerned with energy: its mobility, intensity and apportioning. In a sense then, Freud views the psychic system as one might view a computer. A computer has at its disposal a set amount of energy. This energy is its very lifeblood, yet, in the form of an electricity surge, it is also potentially destructive. For this reason, the computer must both control the overall amount of energy within the system at any given moment (this is the job of adapters and resistors etc.), and, as part of that quantitative control, it must also re-direct the energy to certain sets of circuitry that perform qualitatively different functions. According to Freud, the energy that powers the psychic apparatus is 'libido'. Initially, Freud thought that libido was specifically the energy attached to the sexual instinct, but he later modified this position by arguing that the ego itself had its own store of libido. The economic principle that controls and regulates libido is the so-called 'pleasure principle'. This principle states that, particularly in early life, the individual's psyche is dominated by the pursuit of pleasure coupled with the avoidance of unpleasure. Just as the computer threatens to 'overload' if too much energy is present in its system, so the psychic apparatus experiences excitation in excess of its economic requirements as unpleasurable. In this situation, the excess energy must be used up in some way to stabilise the system as a whole. For Freud, the redeployment of excess psychic energy or libido is achieved by what he terms 'cathexis'. This refers to a kind of electric charge that can be invested in any mental image, idea or structure. For instance, a Christian individual may heavily

[8] Freud, Sigmund. *On Metapsychology* trans. James Strachey (London: Penguin, 1991), pp. 65-97.

[9] Freud, Sigmund. *Beyond the Pleasure Principle and Other Writings* trans. John Reddick (London: Penguin, 2003), pp. 45-102.

'cathect' the object-representation of an apple because a certain quantity of energy has been bound or attached in their unconscious to some perceived sin, or perhaps to a scene of infantile seduction (clearly, this is a culturally specific object-representation). By investing energy in, or 'cathecting', a representation which is only indirectly or symbolically connected to unconscious associations, the psyche as a whole is able to re-direct libidinal energy away from consciousness whilst maintaining the repression of problematic unconscious material.

Four Characteristics of the Unconscious

Clearly, the dynamic, topographic and economic approaches are all intimately interconnected, so much so that is quite difficult to speak of one to the exclusion of the others. In combinations of different emphases however, these approaches allowed Freud to assert the following four primary characteristics of the unconscious:

Exemption from Mutual Contradiction: the unconscious may contain a profusion of instinctual impulses, and many of them may seem in complete contradiction with one another, yet these contrasting impulses do not contradict or diminish one another. Rather, they combine and exist simultaneously so that we may love and hate someone at the same time.

Primary Processes: energy in the unconscious is extremely mobile, which means that, through condensation and displacement, the ideas or images in which libidinal energy is invested can change radically and frequently. The cathexis of the apple in our Christian example above might therefore swap to completely different object-representations, so that, psychically speaking, bananas or cars or cream cakes or really anything can serve the same unconscious function! Only in the secondary processes of the conscious system do 'meanings', or the cathexes invested in them, become more securely affixed to their symbolic representations.

Timelessness: the processes of the unconscious do not recognise temporality in any form, so that from its point of view, an incident which occurred in our early childhood is just as pertinent as one that occurred yesterday or, indeed, five minutes ago. This is acted out by the neurotic, whose symptoms in the present are often defensive reactions to events in the relatively distant past which are nonetheless treated as endlessly new. Time does not heal any of the wounds of the unconscious! Again, it is only the conscious system that imposes temporal orderings, as demonstrated by the phenomenon of 'secondary revision' whereby dreams, in their conscious recollection, are re-arranged into a narrative syntax not actually present in the dream itself.

Replacement of External by Psychic Reality: the unconscious occupies a dark 'depth' far below the bright light of 'reality', so that its processes display a comparative indifference to the exigencies of the outside world. Like an accretion of our residual infancy, the unconscious is dominated by the pleasure principle. This has the consequence that the ideas that circulate in it are governed by their libidinal intensities rather than by their 'meanings' or their relations to objects in reality as such. It is the ego in the realm of the conscious system that tries to impose a 'reality principle' onto the pleasure principle predominant in the unconscious, by directing instinctual satisfactions towards objects and situations in the outside world.

3 Freud: Repression

If the notion of the unconscious is the major 'discovery' of psychoanalysis, the notion of 'repression' is its central explanatory term. Repression is the key to understanding the dynamic approach to the psyche. It immediately suggests the different psychic agencies represented in the topographic approach. It is the very operative law of the economic model. It is utterly indispensable to the therapeutic dimension of psychoanalysis (all symptoms are the result of repression). It is an inextricable component of Freud's theories on the formation and development of the individual subject, particularly in relation to sexuality and, for related reasons, it is the fundamental basis of any psychoanalytic social theory. Moreover, and despite its negative connotations, repression is deemed by psychoanalysis to be a quite normal, and therefore ubiquitous, part of human mental life. In fact, not only is repression actually at the heart of mental *health*, but it is through repression that we come to be who we are.

To understand this crucial concept, we must return to Freud's early analyses of dreams. This is because his primary claim in *The Interpretation of Dreams* – that 'dreams are a form of wish-fulfilment' – involves a close study of the agencies and mechanisms of repression.

The Interpretation of Dreams

On one level, Freud argues that dreams have a very pragmatic, physiological purpose: quite simply, they process internal and external sensations in such a way as to prevent them from waking the dreamer. This is why we dream of fire engines when our alarm clock is going off. However, it is really with the regulation of *internal* or psychical stimuli, such as particularly intense thought processes, that dreams are primarily concerned. Freud's major insight is that the *way* in which dreams regulate these psychic stimuli is meaningful. That we dream at all may be about ensuring uninterrupted sleep, but on another level *what* we dream has a profound psychological meaning for us personally. Dreams, like parapraxes, are not mere nonsense, but have a buried significance which only analysis can reveal.

In fact, the job of regulating these internal psychic stimuli is especially important during sleep. Freud speculates that the control the waking ego normally exerts over the unconscious is weakened during the state of sleep, in which the ego drops its guard. Unconscious desires and wishes contained during wakefulness can therefore irrupt during slumber. Because the unconscious is characterised by powerful levels of libido which often find expression in violent and aggressive thought processes, it is the job of dreams to translate this energy into a different form, so that our own internal thought processes do not wake us up (in this sense, a nightmare is a failed dream). Dreams achieve this domestication of psychic stimuli which are potentially disturbing to sleep by what Freud terms 'hallucinatory satisfaction'. That is to say, unconscious desires that demand a fulfilment that cannot, or rather *should* not, be met with in reality, are appeased by being 'acted out' in a hallucinatory form in dreams. This means that all dreams, no matter how weird or even distressing they are, have at their root an unconscious wish, something we actually *want* to do or have done to us even if we are completely unaware of it. In this sense, dreams are like a safety-valve that lets off unconscious steam by acting out our darkest desires in the much safer haven of a dreamworld, precisely so that we do not carry these into our waking lives, where they would be liable to get us into serious trouble. However, even in our dreamworld this acting out cannot be a literal staging in the form of a direct representation, because the content of the unconscious wish is unpalatable to the conscious (which is still active, albeit in a reduced capacity, during sleep). Freud uses the metaphor of a censor in the mind that the unconscious must get past, deploying disguise and deception to smuggle its wishes into the *Cs.* system.

We can clarify these structures and their relations with a hypothetical scenario. Imagine that during the day you have had a brief disagreement with a friend that seemed insignificant at the time. Imagine, however, that in your unconscious you had immediately begun to formulate an aggressive fantasy about murdering your friend because of this disagreement (remember, the unconscious is by definition an extremely uncivilised place!). Although unaware of them, these thoughts are still swirling around in your unconscious even as your head hits the pillow and you fall asleep. Now, imagine what might happen if, with the decline in the ego's censoring powers as you slip into sleep, this unconscious fantasy leaps into your mind in full and bloody detail. In all probability, you would be shocked into wakefulness, and wonder just where on earth such a strange image had come from! However, now imagine instead that you dreamt you were vigorously chopping a piece of wood with a sharp axe, that with each chop the wood seemed to bleed, and that you experienced a strangely heightened level of satisfaction precisely because of this peculiar bleeding. This might be interpreted as slightly odd, but surely not startling enough to wake you up. This is because the same unconscious fantasy has been expressed in a displaced and distorted way which bypasses the censor. Only with dream-interpretation upon waking might any connection between the argument during the day and the unconscious wish be revealed. Perhaps the surname of the friend you fell out with was 'Greenwood', and this word provided the linguistic pathway for the displaced symbolism of the piece of wood in the dream.

There are therefore at least two agencies at work in dreams, one repressed and the other repressing (just as with parapraxes Freud spoke of disturbing and disturbed intentions). There is an unconscious wish on the one hand and, on the other, some aspect of the conscious that, even in sleep, finds this wish unpalatable. To these two agencies correspond two levels of the dream: the latent and the manifest content. The latent content refers to the unconscious thought processes hidden behind, but at the same time expressed, in a distorted way, in the dream. The manifest content refers to the dream as experienced by the sleeper, or as they recall and report it after waking. Latent content is only accessible by way of analysis. Analysis by free association undoes the distortions of the latent content which went into the production of a manifest content in order to be granted passage into consciousness by the censor.

To use Freud's topographical terminology, an impulse or wish deriving from the *Ucs.* system attempts to force its way into the *Cs.* system. To do so, however, it must pass into the *Pcs.*, which is where such amorphous impulses get assigned symbolic representatives which can be selected by way of some visual resemblance or, as the above example indicated, of some linguistic connection. However, the censor stands at the border between the *Ucs.* and the *Pcs.* systems and will not allow any material through that might disturb the *Cs.* system and therefore interrupt sleep.

As we have already seen, a disguise is required to get past this censor, and enter the *Cs.* system in the form of a hallucinatory fulfilment of that wish. We have already listed these disguises as condensation, displacement, symbolisation and contradiction, but they are important enough to warrant returning to, because they are the basic mechanisms of repression in waking life as well as during sleep.

Condensation describes the fact that the manifest content of a dream seems to be an incredibly compacted version of the much more expansive meanings of the latent dream thoughts, with the dream being the tip of a much larger submerged iceberg. This is achieved by omitting certain elements of the latent thoughts and fusing others into composite figures that stand simultaneously for various things. Freud expresses this well: "A composite figure of this kind may look like A perhaps, but may be dressed like B, may do something that we remember C doing, and at the same time we may know that he is D".[1] It is condensation that makes dream-interpretation so difficult as, because of it, the latent elements of a dream are not substituted in a linear way, with each element being represented by a single new symbol. On the contrary, the effects of condensation mean that any particular dream element can stand for two or more latent thoughts, or complexes of latent thought, or even only a fragment of such thoughts or complexes. In other words, it is condensation that prevents dream-work operating like a simple shift-cipher in an encryption, in which original elements are replaced by other elements selected on the basis of a single

[1] Freud, *Introductory Lectures*, pp. 205-206.

consistent rule. Once its key has been discovered, such a code is as transparent as if there were no code at all, whereas condensation ensures that there can be no single key for explaining a dream because there is no one-to-one relation between its latent and manifest elements.

Displacement is the most obvious and frequent result of dream-censorship. With displacement, some seemingly accidental fragment of the manifest dream *alludes*, in a very indirect way, to the latent thoughts behind it (like the surname of the friend in the above example). Jacques Lacan therefore likens displacement to the rhetorical trope of metonymy, in which a part stands for a whole, as a sail can stand for a ship or a ring for the institution of marriage.[2] In this way, the manifest content is connected to the latent dream-thoughts by only the most remote and twisting path. This is of course in the dream's interests, to the extent that it is engaged in bypassing the censor. Displacement can also operate in waking life, so that the psychic value of a person or activity can be transferred onto another person or activity, with the second becoming a substitute for the first. If you have ever avoided revising for exams by putting excessive time and energy into designing beautifully neat and precise revision timetables, you have engaged in a displacement activity!

Symbolisation can be thought of as the primary representational strategy of displacement, insofar as it enables certain object-presentations to stand for psychic objects that they in no immediate way resemble or evoke (just as the piece of wood symbolised the unfortunate friend in our previous example). Symbolism is necessary if the complex and often abstract nature of the latent thoughts are to be given a *visual* representation which is not transparent or literal for the conscious. Freud gives some long and quite amusing lists of dream symbolism, such as the following, all of which are said to potentially symbolise the 'male reproductive organ' (as Freud was wont to refer to it): sticks, umbrellas, posts, trees, knives, daggers, spears, sabres, rifles, pistols, water-taps, watering-cans, fountains, pencils, pen-holders, nail files, hammers, balloons, flying-machines and zeppelin airships![3] The fact that we experience such lists as comical is, according to Freud, no coincidence. The strange mobility of unconscious symbolism is in direct contrast to the kind of symbolism we are used to in conscious life, when, for example, the capacity of a lion to symbolise courage is more strictly governed by static convention.

Contradiction in the manifest dream content is also far more ambiguous than contradiction as we normally conceive of it in conscious life. Normally, language operates by means of certain binary contraries which mean that when I say 'black' I definitely do not mean 'white' – indeed, this negative, unspoken counter-part is a crucial means by which statements are

[2] Lacan, Jacques. *Écrits*, trans. Bruce Fink (London: Norton, 2006), pp. 412-441.
[3] Freud, *Introductory Lectures*, p. 188.

made. And yet, the world of the unconscious is infinitely stranger. Thus, while 'black' in the manifest dimension of a dream may in fact mean 'black' as it would in everyday communication, it might also mean 'white'! Moreover, and what is far worse, it could also mean 'black *and* white' at one and the same time. This is because the unconscious is characterised by an amazing tolerance for out-and-out contradiction, something the *Cs.* system simply finds baffling. In fact, such a tolerance for contradiction in the unconscious can lead, in our waking lives, to 'ambivalence'. This is a term Freud borrowed from Eugen Bleuler to indicate the simultaneous existence of what, from the point of view of conscious processes, would be considered completely contradictory feelings. Thus, one can simultaneously feel love and hatred towards the same person, just as in dreams the element 'black' can mean 'black *and* white'.

Collectively, the mechanisms of condensation, displacement, symbolisation and contradiction constitute the 'dream-work', which is the distortion of the latent dream content in the interests of getting it past the mind's 'censor' in the form of the manifest dream. In the therapeutic context, the role of the dream analyst is to reverse these distortions of the dream-work in order to try to uncover the latent unconscious thoughts disguised behind the dream as the patient reports it.

Mechanisms of Repression

Having reviewed Freud's thoughts on dreams and the unconscious, let us state the primary characteristics and mechanisms of repression in general, before going on to look at Freud's later complication of the topographic model with the id-ego-superego relation.

The essence of repression lies not in 'getting rid of' or 'erasing' unwelcome psychic material. Rather, it lies in actively turning that material away from a specific region or function within the psychic apparatus: the *Cs.* system that houses our awareness. This 'turning away' is motivated by the pleasure principle, in so far as the psychic material in question would be experienced by the conscious as unpleasurable. In fact, Freud posits two phases of repression: firstly, primal repression and, secondly, what he calls 'repression proper' but which is usually referred to as secondary repression. Primal repression turns away from the conscious the psychic representatives of instinctual impulses. As we have seen, however, the unconscious, like water held back by a dam that searches out cracks and fissures, seeks alternative expression by means of *associated* representations, however distantly derived. Thus, 'repression proper' focuses on these associated representations, actively suppressing the myriad chains of thought and image that might provide a connecting bridge between the *Cs.* and *Ucs.* systems. Put simply, primal repression determines what is unacceptable to the conscious in the first place, while secondary or proper repression denies all the 'ideational' representations (images, words, concepts etc.) by which this unacceptable material might try to force its way into the conscious. And yet, repression is by no means a single event that subdues instinctual representations once and for all. In fact, as Freud says, 'repression demands a persistent expenditure of force, and if this were to cease, the success of the repression would be jeopardized, so that a fresh repression would be necessary'.[4]

Moreover, the targets at which this repressive force is directed are extremely mobile. Not only may an unconscious idea adopt a variety of psychic representatives (images, words, concepts etc.) to try and achieve expression in the conscious, but at any given time that unconscious idea may be attached to different levels of instinctual psychic energy. The possible representatives of that idea therefore require more or less repression in proportion to the energy attached to the idea at that moment. This economic dimension of repression led Freud to speak of the 'quota of affect', which refers to the levels of feeling or emotion attached to an instinct. This is important since it relates to the distinction between, as it were, 'good' and 'bad' repression, which forms the basis of the therapeutic dimension of psychoanalysis. For if repression is governed by the pleasure principle, and hence the avoidance of unpleasure, a repression that transforms an instinct into an affect or feeling which is experienced as *anxiety* should be considered a 'bad' or partially unsuccessful repression. So even though the representative or 'ideational' aspect of an unconscious instinct (the images, words, or concepts which might be associated with it) may be successfully turned away from consciousness, there still may be a considerable amount of *affect* attached to it which is experienced as anxiety or depression. This sounds complicated, but just recall how we can have dreams which seem superficially harmless, yet somehow inspire in us an incongruous dread which is all the more unsettling for having no obvious source in the content of the dream. Freud's distinction between 'psychic representatives' and 'quota of affect' helps to explain this experience. The elements in the dream have been sufficiently distorted for the unconscious idea they represent to remain hidden from consciousness. Yet, from an economic point of view, the 'quota of affect' invested in that unconscious idea still needs to find an outlet, even if it cannot be on the plane of representation, and this is achieved in the form of intense anxiety.

Clearly, this begins to shade into the territory of psychoanalytic therapy. After all, a psychoanalyst's patients will typically have succeeded in pushing unconscious forces completely out of their awareness, yet they will seek help precisely because they feel a general unease, unhappiness, or heightened panic, which has no obvious cause in their external lives. This is

[4] Freud, *On Metapsychology*, p. 151.

when repression threatens to breaks out into neurotic symptoms. From the point of view psychoanalysis, we can say that a symptom is any emotional state, pattern of thought, or mode of behaviour that an individual experiences as abnormal. 'Good' repression is invisible, precisely because it neither impinges on the subject's consciousness, nor emerges in socially unacceptable or bizarre behaviour. In fact, 'good' repression, particularly in the form of sublimation, is the very basis of civilisation and cultural achievement. 'Bad' repression, on the other hand, actually announces its own existence and activities, albeit in strange and misleading ways that impair the individual's social life by breaching generally accepted norms.

So the neurotic symptom is very like a dream, in so far as it represents a compromise between an unconscious wish or instinct and the repressive agency of the ego. However, the 'bad' repression that leads to symptoms is comparable to the 'bad' dream that is the nightmare. For in both cases, the goal of keeping disruptive psychic material away from the conscious leads to compromises which nonetheless rebound upon the conscious in unproductive and distressing ways. What makes the symptom neurotic is therefore that it is a form of repression unserviceable for the goals of normal social life, with which it in fact interferes. The emergence of neurotic behaviour therefore corresponds to what Freud termed a 'return of the repressed'. It is a return because what was deemed unacceptable to the conscious in *primal* repression irrupts into the conscious in the form a breakdown in secondary repression. This leads to an uncontrollable flow of associated representations which the individual still does not understand, even though he or she is acutely aware of the existence of some kind of problem.

The Id, Ego and Super-ego

By the 1920s, Freud was adding further layers of complexity to his theorisation of repression. After coming up against the limitations of his previous theories in trying to explain the neurotic symptoms of his own patients, he introduced a new, tripartite description of the psyche: the id, the ego, and the superego.

The word 'id' comes from Latin and simply means 'it'. In fact, it is an invention of Freud's English translators: Freud originally used the German term *das Es*, and French translators similarly use *ça*. Both phrases convey the sense of an alien or independent entity with an objective reality beyond our subjective control. Both phrases are therefore appropriate, as Freud uses them to refer to a primordial realm that precedes subjectivity and yet forms a crucial part of its dynamics. In many ways, the id is the descendent of the unconscious as Freud had described it in *The Interpretation of Dreams*. Now, however, the emphasis is on the chaotic energy of the instincts and their extremely disordered nature. The id is utterly dominated by the drive to satisfy instinctual needs and, as such, its only law is that of the pleasure principle. It is characterised by violent passions and a primitive disregard for the 'civilised' structures of temporality and logic imposed by the conscious.

In stark contrast, the ego, which modifies the previous term 'the conscious', is an organised realm of the psychic apparatus where the secondary processes hold sway over the primary processes of the id. In fact, the ego emerges from the id as that part of it which is transformed by contact with the outside world. Where the id only recognises the pleasure principle, the ego invents a reality principle by which satisfaction is sought not in hallucinatory fulfilment on the inside, but in 'objects' on the outside. If the id is the realm of passions, the ego is that of reason. If the id is an alien thing, an 'it', the ego is that which we experience as, and call, an 'I'. A whole branch of psychology, called ego-psychology, has arisen since Freud, particularly in America, the therapeutic goal of which is to strengthen the ego. Although some psychoanalysts, such as Jacques Lacan, are critical of this school of thought, it is nonetheless in general conformity with classical psychoanalytical theory because the ego in that theory is essentially defensive, fending off the chaotic aggression of the id on the one hand, and on the other the persecutory voice of the super-ego.

For just as the ego emerges from the id, the super-ego emerges from the ego, as that part of it devoted to self-criticism, and therefore to criticism of the ego where that sense of 'self' originates. The admonitory tone of the super-ego derives from the internalisation of parental figures, particularly the father, who impose notions of right and wrong on the infant. The child absorbs these figures and uses them to police its own behaviour. However, it is not the actual parents that are internalised, but symbols of the parental roles as experienced by the young infant. This means that an actually domineering father may not lead to an individual with a severe super-ego, while conversely, the child of an easy-going liberal father may suffer from acute self-persecution simply because their pre-Oedipal experience of parental intervention led to a particularly aggressive *internal* father figure. This is possible because the super-ego contains numerous unconscious elements. Just as the ego emerges from the id's confrontation with reality, so the super-ego completes the circle, as it were, by also drawing its energy from the id.

In some ways then, the super-ego is a defence mechanism of the ego itself: in order to prevent unconscious aggression being acted out in reality, that aggression is internalised and turned back against the ego. Instead of committing violence against others, violence is committed against the self. Freud's later work therefore recognises that neurotic symptoms do not only derive from the partial repression of sexual instincts, with the ego being attacked from below by the id. This is essentially a dualistic system, with the unconscious and the conscious being the two dominant, albeit antagonistic, systems. Rather, the tripartite division in later Freud helps him to realise that the ego can also be attacked from above, by the super-ego, and that this can lead to specific neuroses such as debilitating guilt and poor self-esteem.

What is new and really quite strange here is that the aggression of the id underlies, indeed fuels, the voice of morality in the form of the super-ego. The tension this invokes between being a 'good' person and self-persecution strongly suggests that the path to moral perfection is fraught with neurotic guilt! This pattern will appear again when we look at Freud's polemic against modern society in *Civilization and its Discontents* in Chapter 5.

4 Freud: Sexuality

If one wanted to demonstrate both Freud's lasting impact on human thought, as well as the *problematic* nature of that impact, one would be hard pushed to pick a better theme than that of sexuality. From his earliest publications, his unusually frank treatment of this topic embroiled him in great controversy, and to this day it remains the focus of the most fervent debates amongst Freudians and anti-Freudians alike.

Alongside *The Interpretation of Dreams*, Freud's *Three Essays on the Theory of Sexuality* can be considered the most influential contribution to human knowledge from classical psychoanalysis. The ongoing importance of the *Three Essays* in Freud's own unfolding thought is evidenced by the number of revisions and rewritings to which he subjected them: first published in German in 1905, Freud was still making additions almost twenty years later in 1924. The three essays referred to address 'the sexual aberrations', 'infantile sexuality' and the 'transformations of puberty'. As ever, Freud was led in these speculations by his clinical practice. He had long noted the heightened tendency towards sexual perversion in his neurotic patients, and it was clinical practice that suggested the existence of the sexual life of children: therapeutic regression had repeatedly indicated that neurotic symptoms were related to the fixation in early life of certain arrangements of the sexual instinct which healthy people 'outgrow'. The *Three Essays* therefore touch positively on the relationship between sexual development and adult normality, and, negatively, on the pathological outcome of an interrupted or discontinuous sexual development. We shall use the first two of these essays as points of entry into Freud's general thoughts on sex and sexuality.

The Sexual Aberrations

It is typical of Freud to start with how things go wrong in order better to comprehend the mechanisms that operate when things go right. Thus, Freud starts his investigation into sexuality by looking at deviations from what is considered normal sexuality. Predictably enough, Freud assumes that normal sexual life involves heterosexual genital intercourse, while sexual aberrations are everything else that affords satisfaction of the sexual instinct.

He divides the aberrations into those governed by the sexual object (or the person we find attractive), and the sexual aim (or the act towards which the sexual instinct tends). The first aberration he deals with is what he calls 'inversion', but which we would call homosexuality – people whose 'object-choice' is of the same biological sex. Freud is actually enlightened enough to be fairly flexible in his account of 'inversion'. He lists three types: absolute inverts (who exclusively choose people of the same sex); amphigenic inverts (whom Freud describes as 'psychosexual hemaphrodites', but whom we might simply refer to as bisexual); and contingent inverts (who, under certain external circumstances and for as long as those circumstances obtain, can take as their sexual object a person of their own sex). Having accepted the existence of such inverts, Freud then sets about trying to explain their occurrence. He dismisses the thesis of degeneracy by which homosexuality was commonly explained away in the Victorian era rather as one might explain a club-foot or a cleft-palette. After all, he notes, 'inverts' exhibit perfectly normal functioning outside the bedroom, and indeed are often 'distinguished by specially high intellectual development and ethical culture'.[1] Here, Freud's apparent liberalism is undoubtedly informed by his bourgeois appreciation of the civilisation of classical Greece, a culture in which great thinkers such as Plato and Socrates openly took young male lovers. He also rejects the argument for the 'innateness' of homosexuality, partly because of the existence of 'contingent inverts' and partly because, even in the case of 'absolute inverts', psychoanalysis often reveals a childhood experience which predisposed them towards same-sex object-choice. He also claims, somewhat controversially from today's perspective, that inversion can be removed by hypnosis!

Nonetheless, Freud isn't satisfied to simply bend the stick in the other direction by arguing that homosexuality is merely *acquired*, since many people are subjected to the same conditions and experiences during childhood, yet only a small number become 'inverts'. Finally, Freud is not happy either with what might seem at first glance to be a psychoanalytic explanation of homosexuality, that is, the theory of 'psychical hemaphroditism'. This theory posits a male and female component within an individual psyche that enables a bisexual disposition. If someone could be physically male, but *psychically* female, it would obviously explain why that person would choose men as their sexual object. However, Freud finds this too simplistic in its reduction of masculinity and femininity to the biological categories of male and female, because, he notes, '[t]here can be no doubt that a large proportion of male inverts retain the mental quality of masculinity, that they possess relatively few of the secondary characters of the opposite sex and that what they look for in their sexual objects are in fact feminine mental traits'.[2] In other words, some gay men want their partners to be feminine, and some gay women want their partners to be masculine. So something else must be going on in the phenomenon of inversion. In fact, Freud ultimately claims that the latter results from the interplay between certain external events during a child's development and

[1] Freud, Sigmund. *On Sexuality*, trans. James Strachey (London: Penguin, 1991), p. 49.
[2] Freud, Sigmund. *On Sexuality*, Penguin: London, 1991, p. 55.

the internal developmental process of sexual maturation. At this stage however, the most important conclusion that we should draw from this discussion of inversion is that *the sexual instinct exists independently of the object towards which the sexual aim tends*: we have desires, and these desires can be directed now towards this object, now that. It is only this surprising mobility of desire, and the substitutability of the objects in which it can be invested, that begins to describe such extreme cases as people who choose animals, or children, or even inanimate objects, as the focus of their erotic instincts.

Having said that, Freud finds the greater number of aberrations in terms of the sexual *aim*, that is, in terms not of who one is attracted to, but in terms of how one obtains sexual satisfaction. Abnormal or perverse sexual aims arise, he argues, from two tendencies: firstly, the tendency to *extend* sexual attention to parts of the body other than the genitals, and secondly, to *linger* over acts, such as kissing, which are usually only preliminary to 'normal' intercourse. Freud's rather rigid definition of the 'normal' sexual aim here, namely heterosexual genital intercourse, threatens to consign just about all of us to the status of perverts! And in fact Freud does warn that the dividing line between perverts and people with 'normal' sexual lives is very slim indeed. Whether one is normal or abnormal rests primarily on the vicissitudes of chance and their interaction with certain constitutional predispositions toward higher or lower levels of libido. Nonetheless, we should not feel too insulted, since Freud also insists that this sexual overvaluation of, and lingering over, non-genital zones of the love-object's body, only becomes fully perverse when those zones are treated *as if they were genitals*.

Nowhere is this clearer than in the case of fetishism, when the zone becomes a complete substitute for genital intercourse.

> What is substituted for the sexual object is some part of the body (such as the foot or hair) which is in general very inappropriate for sexual purposes, or some inanimate object which bears an assignable relation to the person whom it replaces and preferably to that person's sexuality (e.g. a piece of clothing or underlinen).[3]

When a fetishist doesn't even connect the object they fetishise to the person with whom it was originally associated, and particularly when their entire sexual life is contained in their relation to this object – collecting it, touching it, fantasising about it – then one is dealing with a fairly profound perversion (perversion understood, again, as a turning away from heterosexual genital sex). In such cases, the selection of the fetish-object is governed by symbolic relations similar to those which determine the

[3] Freud, *On Sexuality*, p. 66.

specific manifestations of neurotic symptoms, and of the manifest content of dreams. To this extent, the fetish-object can provide a point of entry for the psychoanalytic therapist into the fetishist's particular erotic world, opening up the possibility of exploring the repressed memories of infantile sexual experiences, perhaps even the very experience that led to the later fetishism.

For example, a famous piece of artwork by Meret Oppenheim comes close to being a fetish-object, insofar as it sets up a symbolic relation between an activity centred on the mouth (drinking tea) and a sensory experience which might be provided not only by animal fur, but also by human pubic hair. The implicit reference to oral sex is conveyed here exactly in the manner of an element in a dream, as symbolism and displacement are certainly at work. There is also a humorous dimension which is born of the tonal clash between the civilised associations surrounding tea-drinking, and the sexual act invoked which, as a form of pleasure that does *not* involve heterosexual genital union, is already perverse by Freud's standards.

For a certain kind of fetishist, Oppenheim's visual pun might render manifest how they actually experience teacups (if that is the object they fetishise). Perversions, however, do not only involve inanimate objects. They also involve acts such as voyeurism (what Freud calls 'scopophilia', the love of looking), exhibitionism, the inflicting of pain (sadism), or even the act of receiving pain (masochism). As this ordering immediately suggests, such perversions of the sexual act often come in pairs, so that the exhibitionist is likely also to be a voyeur, and the masochist is likely also to have a sadistic side.

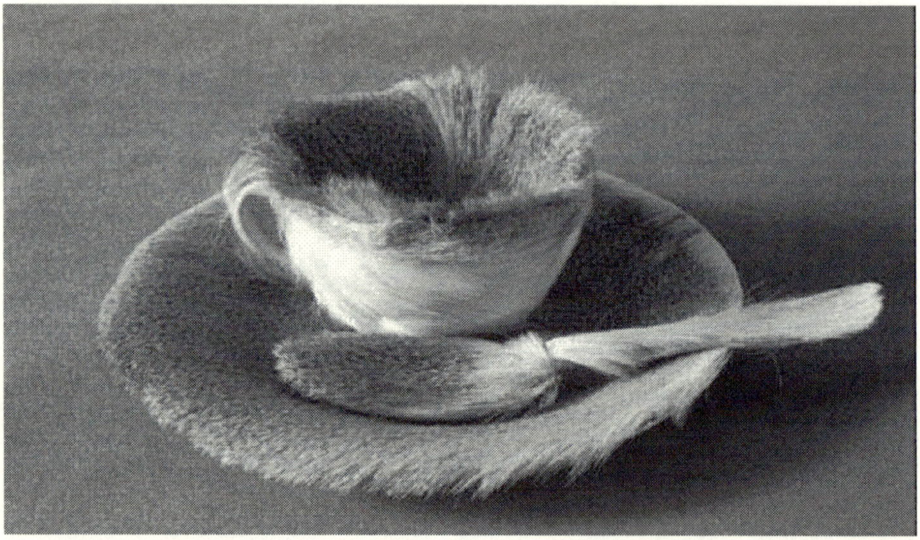

Oppenheim, Meret. *Fur-covered Cup, Saucer and Spoon* (1936).
Overall height 2 ¾ inches. Museum of Modern Art, New York.

It should come as no surprise that Freud contends that there is a close relationship between such perversions and the kind of neuroses psychoanalytic therapy deals with. Indeed, it is as if the two outcomes – perversions and neurotic symptoms – represent opposite responses to the same fixations that can occur during infantile sexual development. Freud's analysis of hysterics had already indicated that their symptoms were evasions of a sexual impulse that they could not face, due to an excessive repulsion for the sexual act. Perversions, on the other hand, represent that same psychic disturbance as it is acted out *within* sexual life, so that neuroses can be considered the negative of perversions. Normal sexual life lies somewhere between these two extremes. Neither carrying over non-genital (and therefore perverse) investments into actual sexual behaviour, nor evading the sexual act by displacing the sexual instinct into neurotic symptoms, normal sexual life is a precarious and fragile thing. It involves channelling that instinct into *heterosexual* object-choice with a view to genital intercourse with such people, at such times, and in such places – and, crucially, in such *ways* – as society is capable of accepting without scandal. On this account, 'normality' in the sexual realm is something of a tightrope which most of us walk with more or less success, but which some of us also chose to flout, secretively in the privacy of our own bedrooms, or publicly in our very lifestyles.

Infantile Sexuality

Freud's most influential contribution to theories of sexuality has arguably been his ideas about the sexuality of children. This was genuinely uncharted territory, and Freud's contributions to mapping it can therefore be considered seminal. In fact, he accounts for the neglect of the sexual life of children in previous writings by arguing that there is a psychological phenomenon called *infantile amnesia* that causes people to forget almost everything prior to their sixth or eighth year. In particular, this amnesia relates to the forgetting of the development of a sexual life up until that point: we have all had infantile sexual experiences, says Freud, but choose not to remember them. Psychoanalytic therapy of neurotic patients subsequently uncovers this amnesia as a form of repression (the memories are there, but turned away from consciousness). However, it is a form of repression common to almost everybody, and this is why most people find the idea of infantile sexuality both abhorrent and improbable.

Nonetheless, Freud claims that the sexual life of children is present from birth, although it only becomes observable at around the ages of three or four. The very fact that Freud imagines newborn babies to have some kind of sexual urge should tell us that he is talking about a very generalised libidinal instinct, rather than, obviously, the act of intercourse. No one would claim that babies yearn to copulate. Yet who could deny that babies are programmed to seek out pleasure, in the form of the mother's breast, and that suckling is a form of pleasure for them? In a sense, this biological drive for the satisfaction of basic desires and the pleasure which follows that satisfaction is Freud's model for the sexual instinct, and it is only later that this same instinct is channelled towards procreation. Survival is at stake in both scenarios: initially for the individual baby, and subsequently for the species in general. Thus, Freud argues that infantile sexuality displays a developmental progression in which various areas of the body (what he calls 'erotogenic zones') succeed one another as substitutes for this initial relationship of the newborn baby to its mother's breast.

However, this progression does not occur in a completely continuous way. It is interrupted by what Freud calls the 'latency period' (a term borrowed from Wilhelm Fliess), during which psychosexual development is stalled until the onset of puberty. Freud is not certain whether this is a physiological or a psychological necessity. However, a strictly psychoanalytic interpretation would emphasise the fact that the latency period generally follows the resolution of the Oedipus Complex, which, as we shall see later, represents a crucial moment in the inauguration of (social) repression. Thus, we can think of the latency period as the result of the repressive demands of parents, who insist that children cease to display sexual behaviour. To hold in check the still extant but now repressed sexual instinct, children during this period develop feelings of disgust, shame and morality unimaginable in the pre-Oedipal phase. This might sound like a wholly negative process, just priggish parents and teachers suppressing children's natural urges. Yet it is more ambivalent than that, as the negative feelings of disgust, shame and moral judgement are also the precondition for *sublimation.* Sublimation is essentially the redirection of sexual instinctual forces away from overtly sexual aims and towards 'higher ideals' connected to the greatest achievements of civilisation: the latency period is, as it were, a rehearsal for this capacity in later life. Yet the period of latency is not guaranteed by some transcendental iron law. External as well as constitutional factors may prevent total suppression of the child's sexuality: they may be subjected to sexual abuse from an adult, or they may simply have a constitutional tendency to a high level of libido which processes of sublimation cannot subdue. Nonetheless, the latency period is a general rule.

But what is the evidence for the existence of the infantile sexuality which latency interrupts? How does it show itself? Well, even before birth (as ultra-sound scans of foetuses in the womb have shown), babies can give themselves a certain amount of pleasure by sucking their thumbs. Clearly, thumb-sucking has no biological purpose (it affords no nutrition). If it does not have that kind of value, then it is likely to have a pleasure-value, a conclusion which is supported by the fact that some people suck their thumbs late into adult life as a way of reassuring themselves. Thumb-sucking actually demonstrates the three main characteristics of infantile sexual behaviour in general.

1. Attachment: it is attached to one of the body's primary functions (in this case, the ingestion of food).
2. Auto-eroticism: it doesn't have an object in the psychoanalytic sense of an external source of instinctual satisfaction, so that it can be described as auto-erotic (the baby is able to give pleasure to itself without help from anybody else).
3. Erotogenic: it focuses on a specific part of the body (in this case, the mouth) which therefore acts as an 'erotogenic zone'.

Some erotogenic zones, such as the genitals and the mouth, are fairly intuitively identifiable, but Freud in fact argues that any part of the body can fulfil this function. This is because infantile sexuality is *polymorphously perverse*, which means that it can take on many forms ('poly' meaning many and 'morph' meaning change), all of which are perverse in the sense of *not* being heterosexual genital intercourse. Infantile sexuality is therefore not centred on any single object or zone, but will seek out pleasure in any form. Once an erotogenic zone becomes established, the child's sexual aim then becomes the stimulation of that zone, although that zone may move. Freud uses these various erotogenic zones to describe both the development of infantile sexuality, and certain core personality types. Here, we come upon a tension in Freud's thought about psychosexual development. For it is not absolutely clear whether he is claiming that the oral, anal, phallic and genital stages (which we shall look at in a moment) are phases that every individual *actually* goes through, or whether he is in fact offering a retrospective description of personality types based on his findings during psychoanalytic therapy.

This ambivalence stems from the fact that these phases were primarily suggested to Freud not by direct observation of children, but by the *accounts* of childhood given during therapeutic regression by neurotic adult patients. Around the issue of infantile sexual development, it is very hard to separate Freud the theorist of sexual normativity, and Freud the theorist of the aetiology of neurotic symptoms. However, the concept of 'fixation' does provide a link between the experience of childhood and later neurotic symptoms. By 'fixation', Freud refers to the tendency for people to over-invest, libidinally, in an object which was only appropriate to a *childish* phase of sexual development but which they have subsequently failed fully to grow out of. In times of stress and psychic turmoil, such people are likely to regress to these fixated forms of sexuality, leading to repeated frustration in adult relationships and even neuroses. If the accounts of Freud's patients are accepted as 'true' revelations of memories previously repressed in the unconscious, then Freud can rightly assert a causal connection between early indicators of infantile sexuality and later personality types and the neuroses to which they are prone. On this account, observing the specific manifestations of sexuality in infants, particularly the erotogenic zones they favour, may actually indicate which neuroses they will become susceptible to upon entering adulthood. Conversely, when, as adults, they seek psychoanalysis, the analyst might be able to refer, backwards as it were, from the patient's particular neurotic symptoms to the probable fixations during infantile sexual development. This is important to grasp, since only in this way can we understand the double role of Freud's theories of sexuality in both his developmental model and his therapeutic framework.

Let us therefore follow the developmental stages asserted by Freud whilst also indicating the personality types to which fixation at such stages can give rise.

Firstly, Freud posits the 'oral stage', which takes place during the first eighteen months of life. Obviously, the erotogenic zone here is the mouth, and the traits of the 'oral' personality include fantasies of incorporation (by which external objects are imagined 'swallowed') and aggressiveness, manifesting itself as biting. Oral personalities are likely to end up being smokers, loquacious talkers, thumb-suckers, or even over-eaters because they obtain pleasure through the mouth. The primary activities of the 'oral stage' are thus to do with a passive receiving and an active taking.

Secondly, Freud posits the 'anal stage', which can last anywhere from eighteen months to between three and five years of age. The erotogenic zone here is the anus. The primordial scene through which to visualise the anal personality is that of the infant stubbornly withholding their faeces, both as a means of asserting control in the face of parental demands ('be good and use the potty'), and to obtain auto-erotic pleasure thereby. In fact, the phrase 'anal retentive' has passed into common parlance, where it is often used to describe someone who is excessively self-controlled. Anal types are the most likely to be misers with money and to hoard things they deem valuable. The activities of the anal personality are dominated by the relationship between giving and withholding, usually with an emphasis on the latter, and also relate to a tendency towards sadism as a means of gaining mastery. On the positive side, this sadistic demand for mastery is also the first stirring of a thirst for knowledge.

Thirdly, psychosexual development enters the 'phallic stage', when, between the ages of about three to five and six to eight, the genitals become the child's dominant erotogenic zones. This is when children are observed to 'play with themselves'. This overt display of a childish sexuality causes particular embarrassment for parents insofar as it is genital, and therefore resembles all too closely *adult* sexuality. Children at the phallic stage are beginning to be aware of the outside world, which had previously been but an extension of their own narcissistic desires, and of the social norms and symbolic systems governing that world. They thus indulge in sexually normative play, acting out gender roles such as 'mummy' and 'daddy'. As their individualised egos are formed in and through this play, they also become aware of other beings as desiring beings with their own love-objects.

The Oedipus Complex

The 'phallic stage' lays the foundations for the famous – or perhaps we should say infamous – Oedipus Complex. This has become a kind of canonical metonym for the whole of Freudian thought, and thus an opportunity to caricature Freud and to dismiss his ideas. Precisely because it lends itself so readily to gross simplification, and yet also because it is in fact a kind of complicated knot which ties together multiple Freudian themes, the Oedipus Complex warrants our close attention.

Its name comes from the Greek tragedy by Sophocles entitled *Oedipus Rex*, in which the eponymous Oedipus is king of Thebes. Oedipus begins the play by trying to find the killer of a man named Laius and to banish that killer from the city. As the play unfolds it emerges that it was in fact Oedipus himself who killed Laius years previously when he had quarrelled with an old man by the roadside on the way to Thebes. Worse, Laius turns out to be Oedipus's own father, who had tried to have Oedipus killed after a prophecy that he (Laius) would be murdered by his own son. Worse still, Oedipus had subsequently married, and had children with, Jocasta, Laius's wife, and his own mother. Oedipus is plunged into emotional turmoil by these revelations, and eventually tears out his own eyes and exiles himself from the very city of which he had been the venerated leader. This ancient Greek drama contains many of the themes which Freud claims occupy the unconscious somewhere between the ages of three and five, when, according to him, boys experience lustful feelings for their mothers.

In fact, one could describe all this in terms of possessiveness – boys simply want to have their mothers, who are after all their primary sources of pleasure, all to themselves. Along with this possessiveness comes jealousy of the person who seems already to possess the mother, and therefore provides an obstacle to the boy's innermost wishes: the father. Hence the unconscious desire to kill the father, 'kill' here operating in the childish sense of 'making gone'. Now, watching children of the age Freud refers to, one can readily agree that the Oedipus Complex could be said to be simply an extreme dramatisation of the natural demand for attention that children so often display. However, there are two deeper similarities between Sophocles' play and what Freud says about the Oedipus Complex. Firstly, in the play, Oedipus spends most of the time completely unaware of his status as the very villain he is trying to track down and banish from

Thebes: this can be thought of as corresponding to the *unconscious* nature of the Oedipus Complex. Secondly, tragic destiny in Greek drama involves human actions being steered, often by the interference of the Gods, towards inevitable outcomes which are not of the individual's own choosing: this can be thought of as the influence of unconscious 'complexes' (Jung's term for a constellation of unconscious ideas) on our everyday behaviour. So even though on one level Freud could be said to be simply dramatising the demand for attention characteristic of every young child as this demand plays itself out between its parental figures, he nonetheless makes deeper claims, on another level, about the interaction between behaviour and *unconscious* forces.

At the stage we have described so far, the Oedipus Complex is simply a stand-off: the boy wants to have the mother all to himself, and he hates his father for standing in the way of this, but because he also fears his father, he is in no position to act on his wish to kill him. This fear of the father arises because of certain banal experiences, such as being deterred from 'playing with himself' by being warned 'I'll chop it off!', as well as finding apparent confirmation of this fear in the sight of female genitalia, which appear to the little boy as a gruesome fulfilment of this threat. These experiences inculcate in the boy what Freud calls 'castration anxiety'. This dread of losing the male member (strictly speaking not castration) is again a dramatisation of the conflict between the sexual instinct on the one hand, and repressive social mores which circumscribe that instinct on the other. Because the Oedipus Complex occurs during the phallic phase, the boy's dominant erotogenic zone is his penis. He is therefore understandably reluctant to have it sliced off by his father, who has already threatened such a cruel act simply in relation to infantile masturbation: how much more likely would daddy be to carry through on that promise were he to discover that his son aspired to steal his wife and, moreover, send him to an early grave!

The boy therefore faces a dilemma: either to continue desiring the mother and live in a constant state of castration anxiety, or to try to repress that desire and identify with the father as the agent of a prohibitive law. Identification with the law of the father at this stage is a precondition for the development of a 'superego', which becomes the *internalised* persecutory voice of the father who represents the wider social mores. The resolution of the Oedipus Complex in this way leads to a series of important consequences:

- the inauguration of sexual repression
- adoption of wider social values as embodied in the (symbolic, not necessarily real) father
- the immediate refusal of infantile sexual life
- entry into the latency period when boys have as little to do with girls as

possible
- and the beginnings of the infantile amnesia, which will mask these traumatic events from adult remembrance

For Freud, this outcome of the Oedipal phase is actually the most desirable, because it is the point at which children give up on their narcissistic and intrinsically anti-social selfishness to embrace the system of values operative in the wider world. In other words, the resolution of the Oedipus Complex is the moment at which children submit to socialisation.

At this point we ought perhaps to underline something which the astute reader should already have noticed, which is that the previous description of the Oedipus Complex applies only to little boys. Little girls are nowhere to be seen, and adult women are present only as objects of desire over which males compete. Indeed, the crucial component of 'castration anxiety' is inapplicable to little girls for obvious physiological reasons. Nonetheless, Freud tries to maintain the integrity of his model of psychosexual development by claiming that girls see their little brother's penises and feel somewhat cheated, insofar as their equivalent organ, the clitoris, is tiny by comparison. According to Freud, they therefore experience penis-envy, and this comes to dominate their adult psychic life as well. It is little wonder that feminists took umbrage at this description! Not only is female sexuality defined negatively by reference to the *absence* of male sexuality, but the simultaneous absence of an equivalent to castration anxiety leads, according to Freud, to a comparatively weaker superego. For Freud, this suffices to explain the moral complacency he imagines to be endemic to the 'weaker sex'. Needless to say, we will be returning to these prickly issues when we consider feminist critiques of Freudian psychoanalysis in Chapter 9.

The final pre-genital stage which follows the resolution of the Oedipus Complex is, as we have already seen, the latency period, which lasts from six or seven to the onset of puberty. This is when the child represses their respective Oedipal attachments and acts out the denial of their own sexuality through a general aversion to the opposite sex. During this stage, boys will play fairly exclusively with boys (deeming boys who flout this unwritten law 'sissies', etc.), and girls, to a lesser extent, will prefer the company of girls. As proof of this period of latency, just ask a child of this age if they have a girlfriend or boyfriend yet, and witness the indignation!

Why the Controversy?

Having looked at Freud's theories of sexuality, we can understand why they are controversial. Firstly, in terms of the initial public reception of psychoanalysis, it is of course predictable that Freud's ideas should meet with moral outrage. Particularly amidst the delicate sensibilities of *fin-de-siècle* bourgeois Europe, speaking about sex at all – regardless of what one said about it – was always likely to incur someone's pious wrath. On a very superficial level then, the response to Freud's work on sexuality was a reaction to the supposedly scientific treatment of a subject generally considered to be beyond the pale. However, it was also the *content* of what Freud said that really caused – indeed, causes – discomfort and derision. The ideas that children have a sexual life, that mothers want babies as a substitute for a penis, and that everybody is constitutively bisexual, seem almost designed to inflame.

To ameliorate this reaction, one could foreground the metaphorical nature of some of Freud's concepts in his discussions of sexual development. When, in speaking of the Oedipus Complex for example, he suggests that the young boy wants to 'sleep' with his mother and 'kill' his father, this is a dramatisation of a libidinal instinct which could just as well be phrased in terms of possessiveness and jealousy – emotions, after all, which are abundantly apparent in all small children (as well as some large adults). The 'wanting' referred to in Oedipal desire is not conscious as such. There can be no clear resolution actually to have intercourse with the mother or kill the father. Indeed, in his comments on the early sexual theories formulated by children themselves, Freud makes it clear that children at the Oedipal stage and long after have no accurate conception of what intercourse actually involves. The notion of 'sleeping with the mother' can therefore only have unconscious and libidinal, not literal, value. But for this very reason we ought to be very cautious about simply invoking metaphor here, as Freud's primary argument is that, precisely as instincts, these 'metaphors' of Oedipal desire are operative in mental life as a genuine and powerful force. Even if it helps to make Freud more palatable to represent his theories as 'metaphors' or just colourful descriptions, one must never forget that these 'metaphors' are at the same time literally real, insofar as they possess an urgent psychic reality.

Moreover, the Oedipus Complex aside, Freud very often literally means what he says about sexuality. He presents infantile sexuality as a biological fact, the existence of non-genital erotogenic zones as a physiological given, and constitutive bisexuality as a psychic reality. Indeed, Freud often expresses astonishment that what are observable facts about sexual life seem to pass completely unnoticed. Predictably, he argues that the repressive force of the ego plays a part in this wilful blindness, and it is this same ego that responds so badly to being confronted with the actual polymorphous reality of sexual life. Again, resistance here confirms the very thing it resists, as the ego – where the conscious resides – is only doing its job *qua* ego in rejecting the wanton impulses of the unconscious.

More important is the controversy *internal* to psychoanalysis, on the part of those who accept the notion of the unconscious and its relation to repression, but do not accept everything Freud said about sexuality. Although in many ways rather enlightened for his time, for example in his refusal to equate homosexuality with degeneracy, Freud nonetheless reinforced many of the prejudices of his era, particularly regarding female sexuality. Indeed, the many feminist critiques of Freud's male chauvinism enable us to view the founding father of psychoanalysis very much as a product of his time. Such critiques encourage us to test the value of his ideas by their capacity to extend *beyond* the limitations of the epoch in which they were formed.

5 Freud: Culture and Society

Culture is a notoriously difficult thing to define. One can think of it, as anthropologists do, as a 'way of life' peculiar to a specific region or group of people; or one can think of it, as Freud tends to, as the body of great achievements within a nation's or a people's intellectual and artistic development. The latter is a rather elitist perspective which one would tend to associate with the upper classes as the predominant consumers of such 'high culture' (working class achievements tend to be conceived of as 'folk culture' or, when mediated by mass consumerism, as 'popular culture'). Yet although Freud as an individual undoubtedly belonged to the bourgeoisie, his notion of culture is far more expansive than just opera, oil painting and ballet. This is because the implications of his psychoanalytic theories pushed Freud's own bourgeois view towards the anthropological perspective on culture. Indeed, culture and cultural achievement in Freud's thought are very closely interwoven with the requirements of society itself. That is to say, whereas even the most ardent advocate of ballet is unlikely to insist that without ballet, society would never come into being, Freud actually does insist that culture – or rather the psychic mechanisms behind cultural achievement – are an absolute prerequisite for social life.

To understand why this is not simply the delusion of a passionate lover of the arts, we shall need to look at the arguments proposed in two very important books written by Freud in 1913 and 1930. These books are, respectively, *Totem and Taboo* and *Civilization and its Discontents*. Juxtaposing these two texts immediately suggests the ways in which an anthropological view of culture overlaps with the elitist or bourgeois view of culture in Freud's later writings.

Totem and Taboo

Written in 1913, *Totem and Taboo* is Freud's foray into anthropology. Anthropology means the 'study of man', and was a particularly flourishing discipline during Freud's lifetime, when, because of colonialism, it coincided with the increasing contact between European and non-European cultures. Colonialism tended to perpetuate the ideology that non-European people were savages who had not yet attained the levels of civilisation found in Europe. This was a useful justification for colonialism, which was seen not as exploitation or oppression but as a benevolent Christian mission to lift the 'backward' peoples of the world from their barbarity. Anthropology seemed to add scientific validity to this notion of 'backwardness', insofar as it both exoticised and infantilised the people it studied. Once again, Freud is rather typical of his Victorian contemporaries in this regard. For just as Freud discovers primitive desires in the sexuality of children which are gradually repressed by socialisation, so he discerns in non-European peoples primitive practices which are gradually repressed by the historical unfolding of civilisation. Thus, in common with the colonial anthropology upon which he draws in such detail in *Totem and Taboo*, Freud views non-European peoples as the 'childhood of humanity'.

Despite the dubious ethics of such a world-view, this approach enables Freud to explore, as stated in his subtitle, 'resemblances between the psychic lives of savages and neurotics'. His fundamental thesis is that neurotic behaviour today finds its precursor in the behaviour of 'savages', either in the past or in other less developed parts of the world. Neuroses are therefore a kind of residue of modern man's (and woman's) primitive past. It is as if Freud is arguing that, beneath our urbane and sophisticated exteriors, the savage that we used to be still lurks in waiting, occasionally irrupting in the form of neurotic symptoms (rather as the demonic Mr Hyde emerges from the intellectual Dr Jekyll in Robert Louis Stevenson's famous novel). However, as we shall see, the similarity between primitive society and the behaviour of neurotics is not an identity: what separates the two – and in Freud's view, separates civilisation from its opposite – is culture itself. For the psychological tensions which primitive men work out in the *social* form of taboos, myths, and religious rituals are displaced by modern man onto sublimated *cultural* forms such as art, literature and science. What 'savages' must control by means of strict and elaborate 'do's-and-don't's' on an external social level, civilised people control by subtle internalised psychic mechanisms. In a sense, then, the juxtaposition of *Totem and Taboo* and *Civilisation and its Discontents* suggests that the prohibitions required for social life precede and enable higher cultural life.

We have already noted that some kind of prohibition is always at the heart of social existence. In *Totem and Taboo*, Freud turns to anthropological work on so-called savages in order to understand what is prohibited in their societies and why, and what forms these prohibitions take. Freud in fact claims that there is one taboo that is universally observable among 'savages', which is that against incest. Immediately, we can detect Freud's interest in investigating the historical origins of the Oedipus Complex and, related to this, the historical origins of civilisation itself. He notes that many anthropologists have commented upon the extraordinary lengths that primitive peoples go to to avoid the danger of incest. Indeed, such is their dread of incest that the very notion is expanded to include not only sexual relations within a family, as we would usually think of it, but sexual relations within a wider *social* unit, such as a tribe or caste.

Thus, drawing on the anthropological work of J. G. Frazer and others, Freud cites the aborigines of Australia. Aboriginal tribes differentiate themselves from each other by reference to a totem, which is usually an animal or a plant or some other object which they treat as a symbol of their founding ancestor, and by extension of themselves. Such totems are not experienced as a mere representation of the tribe, in the way that a flag represents a nation, but rather as the embodiment of the tribe's spiritual essence. So a tribe that believes itself to be descended from, say, a snake god, will venerate and revere actual snakes, to the extent of creating all sorts of taboos (or prohibitions) regarding the touching, naming, general treatment and even depiction of snakes. Killing a snake, whether intentionally or by accident, would be considered by this tribe a heinous crime which might be punishable by death or exile. Thus, totemism necessitates both patterns of shared behaviour (we all treat snakes in the same way) and laws to regulate the breaching of prohibitions (we all know what happens when we *don't* treat snakes properly). These twin demands of ritualised behaviour and collectively observed laws call forth, in their turn, social structures such as the hierarchies implicit between those who conduct and those who participate in rituals, and between those who inflict and those who undergo punishments. The shape of societies springs from this relationship between prohibition and law.

In fact, Freud claims that the most important function of such taboos is to consolidate the *identity* of the tribe in order to differentiate it from other tribes. In our example, members of the snake tribe will always be able to recognise other members of their own tribe by their rituals regarding actual snakes. However, Freud's further claim is that, in underlining tribal identity, totemism actually serves to *regulate the prohibition against incest*, by ensuring that members of the snake clan do not have intercourse with other members of the same clan. Freud calls this 'totem exogamy', which just means that in many of these cultures sexual relations must take place outside the tribe or clan. Originally, this totem exogamy probably had a genuine biological function in the limited gene pool of the tribe's early history (incest in such a situation would eventually lead to congenital deformities), and so was, at that time, closely and openly connected to the incest prohibition. However, this connection becomes forgotten over the course of time. The rituals of totemism come to be observed for their own sake and without *conscious* reference to incest, and these rituals eventually develop into the systems of religious belief we know today. Once again, in suggesting that religions have their origins in incest, Freud demonstrates his peculiar talent for making scandalous assertions.

Perhaps the connection between totemism and the taboo of incest is clearest in the case of what Freud calls 'avoidances'.[1] Freud gives numerous examples of such avoidances. For instance, having reached sexual maturity, boys on Lepers Island in the New Hebrides must leave the maternal home and sleep and eat in a separate dwelling. They cannot re-

[1] Freud, Sigmund. *Totem and Taboo*, trans. A. A. Brill (Harmondsworth: Penguin 1938), p. 28.

enter their maternal home if their sister is there, and if they encounter her by chance she must run away or conceal herself.[2] The Battas of Sumatra regard it as offensive for brothers and sisters to be in each other's company without other people being present, and fathers and mothers will likewise vacate their own houses if they are in danger of being alone with their daughters and sons respectively.[3] Similarly, married men of the African Basogas tribe can only speak to their mother-in-laws if they are in another room and cannot be seen by her, and vice versa.[4] In Freud's eyes, these strangely elaborate rules and regulations which demand that relatives avoid one another indicate an awareness among 'savages' of Oedipal desire. We saw in the last chapter how Freud's theories of psychosexual development suggest that the earliest sexual object-choices tend to be siblings and/or parents, and further that, even after the resolution of the Oedipus Complex, these early choices can be carried over into adult sexuality. Primitive peoples display an acute awareness of these Oedipal forces in their rituals of avoidance.

Moreover, in their meticulous repetition and the dread that attends the very idea of non-observance, the ritual behaviours surrounding taboos closely resemble neurotic symptoms. Obsessional neurotics who feel they must perform certain acts a set number of times, who have phobias about touching certain materials, or who endlessly clean their hands even when there is no rational reason to do so, are not all that different, Freud argues, from primitive peoples who feel compelled to observe certain ceremonies – often themselves involving repetition and ritual cleansing – when confronted by their totem or the breach of the taboos pertaining to it. By making this connection with psychoanalytic theory, Freud is able to relate the psychic dynamics of defence mechanisms to the social mechanisms so obvious in 'savage' societies. That is to say, the economic logic of neurotic symptoms leads to the symptoms themselves becoming the displaced satisfaction of the unconscious instinct they also repress: it is in this way that the obsessive compulsive may eventually derive a kind of libidinal satisfaction from, say, repetitively washing their hands. Freud sums this up succinctly: 'It is a law of neurotic diseases that these obsessive acts serve the impulse more and more and come nearer and nearer to the original and forbidden act'.[5] In a similar way, the rituals and ceremonies of so-called primitive people, and the social structures that arise from them, are built on the mutual complicity between repressed instinctual urges (for example, that of incest) and the prohibitions that regulate them precisely by 'cathecting' them in a very displaced, ritualised form. This kind of feedback loop between desire and its ritualised prohibition will be made

[2] Freud, *Totem and Taboo*, pp. 28-29.
[3] Freud, *Totem and Taboo*, p. 30.
[4] Freud, *Totem and Taboo*, p. 33.
[5] Freud, *Totem and Taboo*, p. 59.

even clearer in *Civilization and Its Discontents*.

In essence, then, Freud's argument proceeds by way of a series of analogies between primitive behaviour and neurotic behaviour that enable him to redescribe the work of anthropologists in terms of psychoanalytic theory. Three main psychoanalytic concepts are brought to bear in this way. They are 'ambivalence', 'projection' and 'narcissism'. We have already seen that ambivalence refers to the maintaining of incompatible yet simultaneous feelings with regard to one and the same object. Now, the very word 'taboo', which is of Polynesian origin but which has its counterpart in most languages, displays this ambivalence, insofar as it can mean both sacred or consecrated *and* dangerous or forbidden.[6] For Freud, this linguistic clue reveals much about the rituals surrounding taboos themselves. Thus, the extreme respect shown by warriors to the enemy, even to the corpses of enemies who have been slain in battle, represents an important concession to the normally taboo breaching of the prohibition, 'thou shalt not kill'. Similarly, the taboo in many cultures around touching powerful rulers may be explained in terms of the ambivalence that leads even loyal subjects to feel intense hostility towards the very leaders they also venerate, rather as Oedipal boys can both love and hate their fathers. The psychoanalytic notion of projection also comes into play in both these examples. Projection is a defence mechanism whereby certain unconscious impulses or wishes are externalised and attributed to other people or things. The warrior who shows respect to his vanquished foe may therefore be projecting onto that foe his own fear of being brutalised by his enemies. The social function of the leader or ruler may be similar to the role of the person who those with delusions of persecution believe are 'out to get them', that is, as a kind of *external* source and cause of all possible evils. Finally, Freud relates these various tendencies in primitive peoples to exactly the kind of primary narcissism he had observed in pre-Oedipal children. Just as primary narcissism refers to the child's love of itself prior to full acceptance of a world beyond its own ego, so primitive societies tend to view external reality, particularly nature in general, as an organic extension of their own tribe or clan. According to Freud, this primary narcissism at the social level explains the widely observed tendency towards animism amongst primitive peoples, which is to say, their tendency to believe that all living things are animated by spirits and have souls and even a consciousness. The notion that trees and plants and animals and even rocks and mountains are vehicles for spirits and demons strikes 'modern man' as absurd and is often dismissed by him as mere superstition, yet Freud argues that such a world-view is quite consistent with the solipsism of primary narcissism.

[6] Freud, *Totem and Taboo*, p. 41.

Civilisation and its Discontents

Writing *Civilization and Its Discontents* some seventeen years later, Freud had had ample time to reflect on the implications of his own findings in *Totem and Taboo.* In the intervening years, two aspects in particular had begun to take on greater importance in his thought: firstly, the prohibition at the heart of social life and, secondly, the way social power feeds on the energy created by its own repressive effects (just as neurotic symptoms can become substitutes for that which they repress). A third factor also comes into play by the time of *Civilization and Its Discontents,* and that is the introduction of a major new concept into Freud's economic terminology. That concept is the so-called 'death instinct' which had been announced in *Beyond the Pleasure Principle* in 1920, and which thenceforward imbued his writings with a bleaker tone, as well as with an even more pronounced dualism.

In *Beyond the Pleasure Principle,* Freud had been forced, by numerous observations made in his clinical practice, to revise his previous thesis that there is a biological tendency towards the avoidance of unpleasure. Essentially, he realised that the pleasure principle alone was not capable of explaining the phenomenon of *repetition* frequently displayed in the therapeutic context, whereby patients would often compulsively re-enact an indisputably negative experience with which only psychic pain, not pleasure, could be associated. This problem was also underlined in the repetitive nature of the dreams of shell-shocked soldiers of the First World War, who insistently dreamt of and had daytime flashbacks to falling bombs even though this renewed the very trauma they suffered from. How could the pleasure principle, which states that the psychic mechanism will always avoid unpleasurable excitation, account for what seems to be an instinct towards precisely pain, loss and even self-destruction? This led Freud to postulate an instinct which somehow pulls living organisms towards a state of absolute equilibrium which is tantamount to their own death, in opposition to the renewal of life sought by the sexual instinct. With his habitual nod towards classical thought, Freud named the elements of this binary between death and creative life force 'Thanatos' and 'Eros' respectively, after the Greek gods of death and sexual love. Although the precise nature of this 'death instinct', or Thanatos, has always been veiled in mystery as well as controversy, and although we shall not be endeavouring to lift that veil here, it nonetheless strongly informs Freud's vision in *Civilization and Its Discontents.*

If *Totem and Taboo* begins to recognise the psychoanalytic mechanisms at work in primitive societies, *Civilization and Its Discontents* represents a passionate polemic against the excessive prohibitions and renunciations demanded by *modern* society. That is to say, despite, or rather because of, their 'backwardness', so-called savages are in some ways closer to an idyllic state of psychological well-being than modern man, who is beset on all sides by the stringent demands of an ever more normative society. While these demands have enabled the pinnacles of human cultural achievement, Freud is uncertain that the price for these achievements has not been a level of misery and neurotic dysfunction that is, from a psychic point of view, considerably too high. In this sense, Freud takes his place alongside thinkers like Karl Marx and Friedrich Nietzsche, who also voiced criticisms of the pathological effects of modernity.

But to understand Freud's particular criticism, we must quickly review the relations existing between repression, libido and neuroses. Essentially, we have said that society fixes the degree of repression that is required to maintain a certain norm, but we have also said that, because of certain constitutional predispositions toward a higher libido, some people find these levels of repression untenable. This leads to libidinal energy being displaced onto neurotic symptoms and therefore to widespread mental ill-health. In other words, it could be said to be society that makes people ill. This is not such a ridiculous idea. After all, many of us would agree that, to some extent, the modern and largely Western phenomenon of eating disorders, such as bulimia and anorexia nervosa, may be related to the norms of physical beauty which society imposes via images in magazines, films and in high-street clothing stores. In this instance, it is clear that society, or at least consumer society, actually makes a profit from the anxieties it induces in the complicity between the fashion industry and the vast weight-loss industry, as well as the health and fitness industry. This example helps us to begin to sense the dialectical relationship between Eros and Thanatos, or libidinal creative energy and an aggressive or self-destructive drive, which is at the heart of Freud's theory of society by the time of *Civilization and Its Discontents*. The anorexic is so concerned to appear beautiful and desirable (Eros) that she practises a form of self-denial that leads, potentially, to death (Thanatos). For Freud, anorexia nervosa could be described as a pathological dramatisation of a structure that is nonetheless essential to social life.

It is in this sense that Freud states that 'it was discovered [by psychoanalysis] that people became neurotic because they could not endure the degree of privation that society imposed on them in the service of its cultural ideals, and it was inferred that a suspension or a substantial reduction of its demands would mean a return to possibilities of happiness'.[7] Insofar as society restricts the freedom of the individual, then, it also threatens to be a source of unfreedom, and therefore unhappiness. The anorexic, for example, is not free to perceive her own body-shape as beautiful on its own merits, but is rendered miserable by the pursuit of an

[7] Freud, Sigmund. *Civilization and Its Discontents*, trans. David McLintock (London: Penguin, 2003), p. 25.

impossible ideal. If it is society that imposes these unhealthy ideals, it is clear that society is operating in a way which few individual members of that society would condone or promote. How many would agree that it is good to have a society that creates unrealistic ideals that lead to mental illness? Yet, arguably, that seems to have occurred. This indicates that society has an agenda of its own which is, potentially at least, in direct contradiction with individual freedom and happiness. A powerful component of that agenda includes creating and maintaining a cohesive social unity by positing 'norms' to which members of that society ought to conform. To be an accepted member of 'consumer society' one must buy certain clothes, listen to certain music, buy one's coffee from certain shops, maintain one's body in a shape which approximates to that valorised in the media, and so on. In a contemporary echo of the tribal scenes invoked in *Totem and Taboo*, modern societies become subtle 'machines' for regulating difference in a network of 'norms', just as, in our previous example, the 'Snake Tribe' set up various prohibitions in order to differentiate itself from other tribes.

The primary point in *Civilization and its Discontents*, however, is that part of the subtlety of such social machines is their psychological acuity. That is, *society exploits the mechanisms of the unconscious in order to create social unity*. As Freud makes clear, it achieves this through careful channelling of libidinal energy:

> [C]ivilisation is not satisfied with the bonds that have so far been conceded to it; it seeks to bind the members of the community libidinally to one another, employing every available means to this end, favouring any path that leads to strong identifications among them, and summoning up the largest possible measure of aim-inhibited libido in order to reinforce the communal bonds with ties of friendship.[8]

To create the energy required for investment in social life, then, a surplus must be created by repressing natural instincts. Aim-inhibited libido is libido deprived of its erotic interest, enabling desexualised social relationships, between friends, between workers and their bosses, between children and their parents, and so on. Fundamental psychic mechanisms such as identification, projection, and of course repression, are all utilised at the level of society to enable individuals to control their narcissistic (or selfish) tendencies. Again, Freud is in agreement with Thomas Hobbes at this point, but he also extends Hobbes's argument. Where Hobbes simply described 'uncivilised' people as intrinsically selfish and vicious, Freud gives a psychoanalytic account of why this should be the case and, more importantly, he also explains why even 'civilised' people are still and

[8] Freud, *Civilization and Its Discontents*, p. 25.

always potentially selfish and vicious. Thanatos, or the death drive, is an instinctual force that tends towards aggression and destructiveness, in the violent expression of which there is an evident narcissistic pleasure (think of wars, of the glory that has always been attached to heroic soldiers and epic battles, and of the apparent fetishisation of the technologies of war today: against the backdrop of the wars which scarred the twentieth century and baptised the twenty-first, Freud's notion of a death drive seems lamentably plausible). Yet for Freud, in contrast to Hobbes, not only does this death drive persist after society has been created, but it is the very source of society's repressive powers. For society is built on the careful redirection of this innate aggression which is the death drive.

> The aggression is introjected, internalized, actually sent back to where it came from; in other words, it is directed against the individual's own ego. There it is taken over by a portion of the ego that sets itself up as the super-ego [...] and is now prepared, as 'conscience', to exercise the same severe aggression against the ego that the latter would have liked to direct towards other individuals.[9]

On this account, unhappiness becomes the lot of the socialised individual. Only those individuals whose super-egos are incessantly stern and judgmental can claim to be 'good', so that 'the very people who have attained the highest degree of saintliness are in the end the ones who accuse themselves of being most sinful'.[10] It is at this point that Freud worries about a dangerous psychic 'loop' which threatens to produce an ever-more accusatory super-ego. For if the super-ego is formed by the renunciation of the drives, and if the super-ego then proceeds to demand *further* renunciations, it frees up more libido upon which to 'feed', thereby adding to its own power through the very exercise of that power! It is this loop that can lead to severe neuroses in which individuals become tormented by their own conscience. This is particularly dangerous when that conscience has grown powerful enough to ignore external reality, and therefore to upbraid the ego on the basis not of thoughts it is actually entertaining, or actions which it has actually endorsed, but on the basis of *imputed* thoughts and actions.

> Whether one has killed one's father or refrained from doing so is not really decisive; in either case one is bound to feel guilty, for the sense of guilt is the expression of the conflict of ambivalence, the unending struggle between Eros and the destructive drive, the death drive.[11]

[9] Freud, *Civilization and Its Discontents*, p. 60.
[10] Freud, *Civilization and Its Discontents*, p. 62.
[11] Freud, *Civilization and Its Discontents*, p. 68.

Some have read this fear of an internalised persecutory guilt as extremely Jewish in tone, yet Freud claims that it is intrinsic to the psychology of all modern social formations. Finding a just and psychologically nourishing form of society is therefore about finding a balance between Eros and Thanatos. Sublimation, as the desexualisation of libido, is the foundation of all the great achievements of mankind. Yet it is also the mirror-image of the aggressiveness of the super-ego, which can lead to a proliferation of neuroses that, in the long run, provide obstacles for civilisation.

6 Jung: the Collective Unconscious

We have now sketched the major tenets of Freudian psychoanalysis. However, this is far from representing a complete account of the movement. While a truly comprehensive account – especially in a small work such as this one – is impossible, we can at least indicate the rich diversity within the psychoanalytic movement by turning now to post-Freudian psychoanalysts. By 'post-Freudian', we do not refer to those who simply came after Freud. Indeed, many 'post-Freudians', such as Alfred Adler, Otto Rank and Melanie Klein, were not only alive during Freud's own lifetime, but were initially his disciples or were at least analysed by him. Rather, the term 'post-Freudian', as used here, indicates those theoretical positions that advance, extend, rearrange, or indeed criticise, Freud's principle insights *whilst maintaining the existence of the unconscious* (this last must be viewed as a defining constant of psychoanalysis in opposition to psychology in general). Considering those who broke away from Freudian orthodoxy also has the virtue of bringing considerable 'colour' to our account, since these apostates were contentious figures who continue to spark heated debates between opposing psychoanalytic camps to this day.

Of no one is this more true than Carl Gustav Jung, the Swiss disciple of Freud who established a version of psychoanalysis which is still *the* rival and antagonist of the Freudian school. An enigmatic and eccentric figure, Jung not only denied some very basic Freudian principles, such as the sexual nature of libido and the dualistic theory of the instincts, but he applied psychoanalysis to previously unrelated realms, such as mythology, alchemy and religious mysticism. His writings are beautiful, yet opaque, suggestive yet, arguably, much less rigorous than Freud's. Even though, in contrast to Freud, he categorically refused to give detailed advice to his followers about clinical practice, there is nonetheless a very distinctive form of Jungian analysis which is practised all around the world today. And, as with Freud, many of his terms have entered into common parlance. For example, the terms 'introvert' and extrovert' are Jungian concepts of which most of us have a basic understanding.

Jung first met the considerably older Freud in Vienna in 1907, a year after they had begun a lively correspondence on the nature of the unconscious. Jung already had seven years of experience in a psychiatric setting at this point, having been first an assistant and then a senior doctor in a clinic in Zurich. He had worked closely with schizophrenics at this clinic, publishing a book on the subject which he had posted to Freud. It is said that Jung was initially bowled over by the already famous Freud on the occasion of their first meeting, and that Freud, in his turn, was immensely impressed with the enigmatic intelligence of Jung (allegedly, their first face-to-face conversation lasted a gruelling thirteen hours). Freud was so impressed, in fact, that, feeling a gentile would be better placed to disseminate what was already being reductively labelled a 'Jewish Science', he elected Jung the first president of the International Psychoanalytic Association in 1909, and made him editor of the world's first psychoanalytic journal.[1]

Always extremely careful to ensure and control his legacy, Freud had earmarked Jung as his heir apparent very early on. Yet his plans soon went awry, as a personal as well as a theoretical chasm opened between the two ambitious men. Travelling by ship to lecture in America in 1909, both men passed the time at sea by analysing one another. Unfortunately, Jung was frustrated by the resistance which Freud himself seemed to be showing to analysis, while Freud, for his part, quickly discerned an Oedipal relation in which Jung entertained patricidal unconscious intentions towards Freud as the figurative father of psychoanalysis! One hardly requires acute psychoanalytic insight here to speculate that burning jealousy, on both sides, was destroying their friendship. By 1913, Jung had resigned as editor of the *Jahrbuch*, and the following year he withdrew from the International Psychoanalytic Association altogether, pointing out that 'my views are in such sharp contrast to the views of the majority of the members of our Association that I can no longer consider myself a suitable personality to be president'.[2] While Jung had already shown a flair for independent thought, this personal split with Freud and with Freudianism undoubtedly motivated his subsequent articulation of an explicitly *anti*-Freudian psychoanalysis.

The divergences between Jungian and Freudian psychoanalysis are complex and legion, but here we shall confine ourselves to fundamental or overarching differences in just three important areas:

1. The Unconscious
2. The Sexual Theory of Libido
3. Personality Types

The Collective Unconscious

Superficially, Jung's tripartite division of the psyche looks a lot like Freud's own early postulation, in *The Interpretation of Dreams*, of a conscious, a pre-conscious and an unconscious system. Jung's very terms invite this comparison, for he speaks of a 'conscious', a 'personal conscious', and a 'collective unconscious'. However, as always with Jung, we have to be wary of what translators call *faux amis*, or 'false friends' (words that look like they have obvious equivalents, but do not). While the

[1] Namely, the *Jahrbuch für Psychoanalytische und Psycho-pathologische Forschungen*.

[2] McGuire, William (ed.). *The Freud/Jung Letters: the Correspondence Between Sigmund Freud and C. G. Jung* (London: Hogarth Press, 1974), p. 551.

Jungian conscious is essentially similar to the Freudian conscious, the personal conscious in no way corresponds to the Freudian pre-conscious. Early Freud argued that the pre-conscious is the system that filters symbolic derivatives coming from the unconscious into the conscious, repelling associations which might trace a pathway back to repressed material. For Jung, in contrast, the personal conscious is seemingly closer to the Freudian *un*conscious in that it is the storehouse for repressed, forgotten or simply latent psychic elements which are not yet ready to enter the conscious system. It is specifically designated as a 'personal' unconscious, however, because it is acquired over time by the individual subject, and is unique to them. In contrast, Jung claims to have discovered a *collective* unconscious which is at a deeper layer of the psyche than Freud ever managed to explore, the contents of which are not specific to the individual subject, but are rather an *inheritance common to the whole of humanity*.

This strange idea evolved from Jung's earliest work with schizophrenics. Freud had long declared schizophrenia to be off limits to psychoanalytic therapy, since sufferers were incapable of the transference required to work through their unconscious complexes. Jung was the first psychoanalyst to argue that the bizarre and seemingly impenetrable discourse of schizophrenics was not simply nonsense, but was in fact meaningful, albeit in a way totally estranged from everyday speech. In fact, he found that one could only explain the erratic expression of schizophrenics by leaving their personal histories behind. Instead, the therapist had to delve into the archaic motifs and primordial images which appear again and again in the symbolism of the world's mythologies and religious systems, and which, according to Jung, also crop up in schizophrenic discourse. Something about madness, claimed Jung, tapped into a psychic reservoir of universal unconscious symbols.

In a sense, with this notion of the 'collective unconscious' Jung is pursuing to its absolute limit a possibility already raised by Freud himself. As we have seen, in *Totem and Taboo*, Freud makes a very explicit connection between primitive tribal social systems and the nature of the unconscious today. This linkage implied that psychological reality may be something like a sedimented archaeology, with the past being retained in the present but in a deeply buried form. Jung simply took this notion of the unconscious as a repository of the primitive past and asked whether there might not be such a thing as a collective (unconscious) memory of this past which could affect the individual but without being reducible to his or her own personal experience. Although he was speaking more in biological than in quasi-mystical terms, Freud had already made the argument that there are both phylogenic and ontogenic components to psychosexual development, pertaining to the level of the species and the individual respectively. Jung radicalised the phylogenic dimension and paid little attention to the ontogenic aspects of individual development. The collective unconscious, at its darkest depths, is in fact incomprehensible to the individual ego precisely because its elemental force transcends individual experience.

Another way to look at this issue would be through the Oedipus Complex. Freud used Sophocles' play in an apparently allegorical way to describe the contents of certain infantile unconscious fantasies: the little boy's ambivalent hatred for his father was *like* Oedipus' albeit inadvertent murder of his father. However, Jung speculated that the relation between Greek mythology and the contents of the unconscious might not be allegorical at all, but quite literal! Why, he asked, does a two thousand year old myth from another epoch and another culture describe so perfectly the psychic structures which Freud, an Austrian Jew at the turn of the nineteenth century, was claiming to have discovered for the first time? Was this pure coincidence, or was this because both Sophocles and Freud were dipping into an almost timeless realm that we all have in common: a collective unconscious?

One can therefore consider the collective unconscious on two levels, the biological and the cultural. On the phylogenic or biological level, the collective unconscious is like a kind of DNA of the psyche: just as DNA is a structure common to all organic life, so the collective unconscious is hard-wired into the structures of the brain. Just as DNA is made up of a relatively small number of constituent elements that nonetheless account for the dazzling profusion of forms of organic life, so the collective unconscious has a restricted number of psychic elements that nonetheless produce the infinite shades of mental life that we are capable of experiencing. But on the cultural level, too, the collective unconscious has provided images and ideas which inspire forms of expression across the world: religions, mythologies, fairy tales and even literature and painting from all regions and all epochs therefore provide, according to Jungians, a kind of aesthetic record of the universal existence of the collective unconscious. Jung himself travelled extensively to places like India and Latin America, and conducted intensive research into Eastern art forms and religious systems, in order to search for traces of the collective unconscious in the traditions of non-European cultures.

But how does this collective unconscious manifest itself in everyday life? Jung claimed that there are certain primordial structures of thought which come from the collective unconscious and which he called 'archetypes'. These produce images and emotions which he described as 'archetypal', i.e., symbolic representations of the archetypes whose existence can only be inferred from these representations. Such archetypal images could crop up in dreams, in the visions of mystics, in the babbling of schizophrenics, or just in everyday fantasies. For example, we might dream of an elderly gentleman who seems to have something important to say to us. Where a Freudian is likely to begin talking of father-complexes, a Jungian might see this as an archetypal image of the Wise Old Man, a figure common to nearly all mythologies and fairytales (think of King Solomon in the Bible, or the legend of Merlin, or Gandalf in Tolkien's *Lord of the Rings*). This archetype might be interpreted to mean that the dreamer is feeling confused and looking for sage advice. Archetypes are thus not intrinsically pathological, but common to us all, irrespective of our state of mental health. Indeed, Jung sees the archetypes not as products of a fundamentally aggressive unconscious as Freud's later work, influenced by the notion of the death drive, had started to describe, but as potentially positive guides for individual behaviour – the Wise Old Man mentioned above might be able to provide actual psychic assistance.

So where Freud suggested that neurotics are the last people to understand their own neuroses because of the effects of repression, Jung felt that individuals always carry the solutions to their own psychological problems within themselves. Indeed, the archetypal images arising from their own unconscious could show them the way towards self-healing. The role of analysis is thus to reveal to the patient what, at some deep level, they already know. Jungian analysis therefore centres primarily on the identification of 'archetypes' and the specific therapeutic potential of those archetypes within the symbolic systems of which the patient is a part: family, friends, nation, even world. In this sense, it is obvious why Jung should be so much more sympathetic to religion than Freud. Whereas Freud considered religion to be an illusion born of projections of the internalised voice of the father in the form of the super-ego, Jung looked upon religion as a body of knowledge in which the symbolic grammar of the archetypes had been carefully collated. He was particularly interested in accounts of the visions of religious mystics because he interpreted them as extreme forms of self-administered therapy in which individuals had delved deep into the collective unconscious in order to retrieve a kind of archaic wisdom. Indeed, Jung, like Freud, was a critic of the pathologies of modernity, insofar as he felt that this archaic wisdom evidenced by the traces of the archetypes in mythology, religion, folklore and so on, could provide a corrective to the alienation and creative stagnation of modern life, but was being lost amidst a misplaced and rather arrogant faith in science and scientific rationality.

Perhaps on the model of the reclusive religious mystic (which he himself embodied at various points in his life), Jung posited as *the* goal for psychological health what he called 'individuation'. This term refers to the process of psychological differentiation, that is, of distinguishing the self from others by developing an individual personality. This is different from Freud's notion of 'maturity', which always implied adherence to socially acceptable norms. Jung, who is generally less prescriptive, argued that even the most isolated, eccentric individual could be well individuated in the sense that they could be aware of their own unique psychological reality.

Jung is no ego-psychologist, however: individuation is not simply a matter of bringing the ego into consciousness. On the contrary, individuation involves accepting one's strengths *and* one's weaknesses as part and parcel of a whole psychic system that is in turn part of wider social systems. This means that individuation is not about getting to know oneself in isolation, but rather, it is about getting to know oneself in one's condition of perpetual indebtedness to others. To this extent, it is possible to discern in Jung's notion of 'individuation' quite a humanist tone.

The Sexual Theory of Libido

One thing everyone knows or thinks they know about Freud is that he saw sex at work behind everything. While our comments in the previous section on sexuality will have clarified that Freud is in fact concerned with a very basic drive which can in no way be reduced to the act of sexual intercourse, it is certainly true that what Freud calls 'libido' is described as the decisive force behind all mental activity. The sexual *instinct* then – thought of as the pursuit of pleasure rather than of one particular source of that pleasure in sex conventionally understood – is indeed the energy that gives the Freudian psychic apparatus both its dynamism and its coherence. To deny the centrality of the sexual instinct is really to challenge the entire explanatory power of Freudianism. Yet this is exactly what Carl Jung did.

The point of no return in the split between Freud and Jung occurred during another series of lectures in America in 1912. Speaking at Fordham University in New York, Jung claimed that an exclusively sexual theory of libido was inadequate for understanding the more psychotic complaints such as schizophrenia, thereby suggesting a limitation of the Freudian approach. So while Jung agreed with Freud's interpretation of hysteria and obsessive compulsive disorders as essentially sexual in nature, he refused to endorse the idea that libido in general was necessarily sexual. Indeed, Jung began to suspect that Freud had unjustifiably projected adult reproductive sexuality backwards onto infantile development, mistaking basic physiological drives like hunger, thirst and the need for sleep for erotic relations. At a stroke, this casts doubt on Freud's complicated narrative of psychosexual development which is also the foundation both of his theories of personality types and, with the concept of 'fixation', of regression as a fundamental principle of Freudian therapeutics.

Inevitably, this disagreement over the nature of libido led Jung and Freud to clash on the thorny issue of the Oedipus Complex. As we have seen, incest is an absolutely central part of Freud's explanation of that complex: the boy, albeit unconsciously, lusts after his mother. If Jung was right that Freud overestimated the importance of sexuality, this surely would be the place to prove it! In fact, Jung simply interprets the Oedipus Complex differently. Where Freud sees an incestuous relation to the actual mother, or at least to her psychic representative in the child's mind, Jung sees an archetypal image of the *universal* Mother. The apparent aggressive possessiveness towards her is in fact an attempt to 'return to the womb', or to return to the security of infancy, particularly at times in the subject's life when their circumstances are providing a challenge to which they must adapt. In other words, when things get tough, we tend to react by wanting to return to a past of supposed wholeness and unity, and it is then that the collective unconscious proffers incestuous symbolism as the invocation of a re-union, rather than a coupling, with the mother. According to Jung then, the Oedipus Complex is therefore nothing but a variant of very ancient 'Sun Myths' found in cultures around the world, from the ancient Egyptians to the druids who built Stonehenge, from the Aztecs to the Aborigines. In such myths, the archetype of the Sun is very often connected to that of the Mother because of their common connection to fertility: the sun 'gives birth' to the crops people need to survive, just as mothers give birth to children. In contexts of scarcity then, neither good harvests nor healthy offspring can be assured, so that the daily dawning of the sun is seen as a miraculous process of re-birth marked by a kind of divine benevolence, rather than by the metronomic certainty of a Copernican view of the universe (in which we *know* the sun will rise tomorrow, irrespective of our prayers). Here we can see how the collective unconscious, in drawing on these Sun Myths, both expresses a psychological dilemma and indicates a possible positive solution. The Oedipal child is faced by problems to which he must adapt but to which he initially reacts by fantasising about a regression to a time free of problems and responsibility. And yet, in the archetypal symbolism of re-birth, it is also possible to see the wished for 'return to the womb' as a new start, and therefore as a fresh take on the dilemma motivating this complex.

But if it was not exclusively sexual, what was libido according to Jung? In many ways, and like many Jungian concepts, the answer to this is frustratingly general: Jung expanded libido to encompass psychic energy in general. Any thought, image, expression or behaviour in psychic life is evidence of a libidinous force. While he retains the notion of desire, this is no longer in any simplistically sexual sense, but rather in the sense of 'appetite in its natural state'.[3] This idea of a 'natural' state is important, because it signifies the direction of a flow of energy when left to its own devices, unmolested by prohibitive moral authorities. If there are no immediate repercussions in eating a cream-cake, our libido will always lead us to do so! For Jung, this has nothing intrinsically to do with sex. It is natural in the same way that water, poured onto a gradient, will always flow

[3] Jung, C. G., *Complete Works, Volume 5 – Symbols of Transformation: An Analysis of the Prelude to a Case of Schizophrenia* (London: Routledge, 1967), para. 194.

downhill. This is the sense in which Jung speaks of 'finality', as the tendency of all psychic activity to gravitate towards a potential result: 'The flow of energy has a definite direction (goal) in that it follows the gradient of potential in a way that cannot be reversed'.[4] The libido becomes a positive and creative life-force immanent in all psychic activity. Indeed, at moments, Jung seems to return to a kind of animism whereby libido is *the* life-force, subjective or objective, rather as the philosopher Spinoza posits a divine substance behind all life.

At this point, Freudians protest that Jungian psychoanalysis posits a monistic theory of the libido that completely flattens all of Freud's dynamic claims regarding the tussles between Id, Ego and Super-ego, as well as between Thanatos and Eros, and to that extent forecloses economic aetiologies of neurotic complaints. In fact Jung does have a theory of the economics of the psyche, although it is much simpler than Freud's. Instead of a complex dialectic between life and death drives, he proposes a mechanism of *compensation* whereby the psyche, which naturally aims at harmony and wholeness, tries to maintain a balance between levels of libido in the conscious and unconscious systems. This is exactly like the balancing of scales, where the two sides are the conscious and the unconscious. The psyche is a self-regulating system with consistent levels of libido, so that the same amount of 'weight' needs to be distributed between the two axes in whatever permutations enable equilibrium. In neuroses like depression, it appears as if there has been a diminution of libido – the subject is physically lethargic, and is difficult to motivate – and this might seem as if some of the 'weights' have been removed from the psychic scale altogether. However, in the depressive state the libido has merely retreated from sight, so that the amount of libido is the same, but the scales are now overbalanced on the side of the unconscious. For the invisible libido has regressed into the unconscious to delve into the resources of archetypal symbolism in order to *compensate* for destructive attitudes in the conscious (such as low self-esteem). The job of analysis is then to aid the subject's individuation by bringing to consciousness, through dream-analysis, free-association, art therapy and so on, the archetypal symbols toward which the libido is turning. In theory, this should balance the scales of the psyche between the conscious and the unconscious, which must be the goal of mental health.

Personality Types

This relative desexualisation of libido in Jung's thought also had

[4] Jung, C. G., *Complete Works, Volume 8 – The Structure and Dynamics of the Psyche* (London: Routledge, 2000), para. 2f.

implications for the Freudian theory of personality types. First, what are personality types? Well, the psychology of personality types is somewhat reductive insofar as it attempts to fit individuals into pre-existing categories that can be useful in determining therapeutic approaches. That is, if the therapist can identify a patient as a hysterical personality type, this immediately indicates a way of treating them. While this may tend towards the effacement of individual differences, of what makes the patient unique, many therapists find it a useful guide in their clinical practice. After all, this is generally how medical diagnoses work. As the example of the hysterical type shows, one way of approaching personality types is to describe individuals in terms of the neurotic conditions towards which their behaviour and outlook predisposes them (although this does not mean that they must actually be neurotic). So such clinical personality types would include, as well as hysterical types, also manic, obsessional, schizoid and phobic types. This means that while someone may not show evidence of neurotic compulsions, their meticulous, tidy, well-ordered and controlling behaviour may be aptly described under the heading of 'obsessional'. This would be the clinical approach to personality types. However, as we saw in relation to the *Three Essays on Sexuality*, Freud combined this with a developmental approach. In those essays, Freud proposed four personality types which were linked to libidinal (sexual) development: the oral, anal, phallic and genital types. For Freudians, the fixation of libidinal formations at particular stages of psychosexual development can lead to a regression back to these pre-Oedipal formations in later life, thereby stalling normal sexual development and creating the conditions for neurotic symptoms. Specifically, the character traits associated with these developmental stages (oral passivity, anal sadism, phallic compulsiveness and so on), are exacerbated by the regression to fixated libidinal arrangements. In this sense, Freud combines the clinical and developmental approach to personality types.

As ever, Jung paid much less attention to the developmental dimension, although his particular notion of libido was still central to his theory of personality types. Before we go on to look at this theory, however, we should mention an important distinction that Jung introduced which is not really to be found in Freud (although his 'ego-ideal' might be considered approximate). That distinction is the one between 'personality' and 'persona'. As we have already seen with 'individuation', Jungian conceptions of personality involve a process of differentiation, with the individual becoming aware of his or her distinction from, but also location in, the values and norms of the society he or she lives in. Personality represents a kind of Darwinian adaptation which 'naturally' selects the psychological formation most appropriate to the demands of the individual on the one hand, and the society in which they find themselves on the other. In a sense, the 'persona' is one strategy within this overall personality, although it is one with implicit dangers. The word persona literally means 'mask', and this really describes its primary meaning in Jung, because he uses it to refer to the outward facing identity that we present to the world, which may well help us make our way through that world, but which is not really part of us. Most of us can grasp this notion of the persona quite easily. Imagine being at a party and feeling unsociable but 'putting on a friendly face' anyway. This outward presentation of something we do not really feel can, as in this instance, make social interactions much more successful. Where do we get these personae from? Well, it is certainly not from within ourselves! Invariably, personae come from the outside, in today's world from ideals in the broader media. For example, we may look at the world relatively early on and take note of the fact that pop stars seem to receive great adulation. We might decide that it would be nice to get some of that attention, so we might take on, and project to the outside world, the persona of a high-profile celebrity. We might be so proficient at this that we end up living our dream and becoming an actual pop star. However, this is where the persona can also become the source of neuroses, because this projection of an ideal never really fitted with our true individuality. Without undergoing successful individuation, which is in part the differentiation of the persona from the ego, we can become trapped by our own personae.

So Jung is careful to point out that, before even examining personality types, one has to get beyond the projected persona. Once beyond that point, argues Jung, a typology of personalities must consider the unique play between what he calls 'attitudes' and 'functions', and the ways in which these effect the movement of libido. Attitudes denote an individual's predisposition to react to events in a certain way, while functions are *means* of reacting. Attitudes result from the predominance in any given individual of any one of four functions that Jung identifies: sensation, thinking, feeling and intuition. He explains these as follows:

> Sensation establishes what is actually present, thinking enables us to recognize its meaning, feeling tells us its value, and intuition points to possibilities as to whence it came and whither it is going in a given situation.[5]

Most of us have these four psychological functions, but we invariably favour one over the other, and favouring one to the exclusion of the other three is likely to result in neuroses. When combined with an assessment of the direction of the flow of libidinal energy, functions and their interaction with attitudes enabled Jung to distinguish eight personality types which are

[5] Jung, C. G., *Complete Works, Volume 6 – Civilization in Transition* (London: Routledge and Kegan Paul, 1970), para. 958.

really very different from those which arose from Freud's sexual theory of libido. The two fundamental personality attitudes are 'introverted' and 'extroverted', and these interact with the four functions of sensation, thinking, feeling and intuition, but with each of these functions having their own introverted or extroverted tendencies. Introversion and extroversion can easily be understood in terms of the direction of libido, whether it flows, respectively, into the inner world of the instinctively private individual, or outwards towards the 'outside' world. Introverts are rather shy and retiring, perhaps even a little defensive. They will shrink back from certain exterior events and put great store by private reflection and thought. Extroverts, by contrast, are gregarious and outgoing. They will adapt quickly to exterior events and will value action and decisiveness. The two attitudes emphasise the subject and the object respectively. Jung's goal was not to set up a normative hierarchy of better and worse personality types. Indeed, Jung claims that we all have all eight of these 'types' within us but for various environmental and historical reasons we generally emphasise one above all others. However, this lop-sided emphasis can change, and his therapeutic stress is therefore on a holistic approach which encourages the deployment of all eight personality types in the situations for which they are most appropriate.

Another very big difference between Freudian and Jungian theories of personality is Jung's (from a Freudian perspective very bizarre) habit of giving the unconscious itself a personality! Whereas for Freud the personality is really the exclusive province of the ego, for Jung, the unconscious has its own character traits. Indeed, these traits are explicitly gendered. Thus, the 'anima' is an archetypal image of woman that betrays the feminine side of the male psyche, and serves not only to balance the aggressively male 'persona' but also to mediate his relations with actual women. Clearly, this notion is indebted to Jung's other presupposition that the unconscious always compensates for what is going on in the conscious, including gender roles. So a macho and tyrannical persona will be compensated for by an unconscious anima that is feminine and sensitive, and furthermore this tyrant will project this ideal woman onto actual women and become besotted with women who seem to embody the anima's qualities. Conversely, the 'animus' is an archetypal image of man that betrays the masculine side of the female psyche. So a woman whose animus is attempting to compensate for her conscious may become ultra-rational and convinced of the infallibility of her own reasoning, and again she is likely to view actual men in her life through a haze of stereotypes and prejudices which actually come from the collective unconscious.

Irreconcilable Differences?

So are Jung and Freud destined to be forever at loggerheads? Must Jungians and Freudians still cross the road to avoid one another? Or can there by some kind of rapprochement? In fact, since the very personal and very public split between Jung and Freud, much water has passed under the bridge of psychology. Firstly, psychoanalysis in general is much less dominant in psychology, which now tends to be behavioural in approach (negative patterns are put down to maladaptive learned behaviours rather than to the influences of an unconscious). But secondly, in the clinical context, many psychoanalytic therapists have found ways to use Freudian and Jungian forms of analyses in conjunction with one another. In particular, many have supplemented Freud's incisive scientific terminology with Jung's more holistic approach which considers patients in their wider personal contexts. The doctrinal differences between the two psychoanalytic theories have proven more intractable on the abstract level than have therapeutic collaborations on the practical clinical level. Sándor Ferenczi's quip that 'the Jung no longer believe in Freud', while still amusing, is perhaps less applicable today.

7 Klein: Child's Play

Unlike Jung, Melanie Klein never deliberately repudiated Freudianism. Despite the dramatically new direction she opened up for psychoanalysis, she and her followers always characterised this direction as a deepening and extending of the trajectory initiated by Freud himself. Nonetheless, like Jung, her ideas met with fierce resistance in some quarters. Indeed, a very heated and public argument between Klein and Freud's own daughter, Anna (herself a psychoanalyst), led to a theoretical split between British and continental approaches to psychoanalysis.

In some ways, Klein's background was similar to Sigmund Freud's. She too was born in Vienna (in 1882), and she too came from a middle-class Jewish family (her father, Moriz, was a doctor). However, there was an obvious difference that was significant at this time: Klein was a woman. As a woman, her own medical ambitions were initially stifled by marriage and then motherhood. When she finally came to psychoanalysis, it was relatively late in life. Only in 1914, already thirty-two years of age and a mother of three, did Klein suffer the bout of post-natal depression which led her to undertake therapy, in Budapest, with the Hungarian analyst, Sándor Ferenczi. This encounter with psychoanalysis as a patient was a revelation, inspiring her to renew her intellectual aspirations by grappling with Freud's theories. Ferenczi supported this decision, and, perhaps because it fitted with prevailing stereotypes about women, but also because it was an area of his own interest, he encouraged Klein to work with children. He appointed her as a clinical assistant at his own Association of Child Research, and was delighted to see, in 1919, the former patient become an analyst herself. As a woman in an extremely male-dominated profession who also lacked formal medical training or indeed an advanced degree of any kind, Klein's personal achievements were already considerable.

But just like 'career women' today, Klein found it difficult to reconcile this new profession with her family life and, perhaps inevitably, her marriage crumbled in 1921. Soon afterwards, she moved to Berlin, where she sought to continue her analysis, now with Karl Abraham, who would also influence both her thought and her career (notions of introjection, for example, are very important in Kleinian theory, which was something she learnt from Abraham). Flourishing under these influences and liberated by her divorce, Klein immediately set about making original and substantial contributions to theories of childhood development and fantasy life. On the strength of her growing reputation, she was invited in 1925 to give a series of lectures in Britain, where child analysis was already a vibrant area of research and where – again not coincidentally – many women belonged to the British Psycho-Analytic Society. These lectures were a *tour de force* and, in 1926, Ernest Jones invited Klein to move to London and live in Britain permanently. She accepted, and the theories she came to develop through the observation of young children went on to exert a profound influence on the way psychoanalysis would be conducted in Britain.

Thus, although Klein, like Freud, was Austrian, her name is now indelibly associated with a specifically British school of psychoanalysis. Nonetheless, her influence has now stretched far beyond the shores of the British Isles. Klein radically revised orthodox Freudianism, extending its therapeutic application to very young children, schizophrenics and even to the psychologies of groups. Her emphasis on the importance of the mother in processes of subject-formation has also left an important legacy to psychoanalytic feminisms.

Child Analysis

Klein was not the first person to analyse children. This honour goes to Freud himself. For example, Freud famously analysed the anxious behaviour of 'Little Hans', a five year old boy whose incipient agoraphobia expressed itself as an irrational fear of being bitten by a horse. According to Freud, the horse was displaced symbolism pertaining to Hans's own father, and the attendant fear was a form of castration-anxiety typical of the Oedipal phase. Freud also analysed the behaviour of his own grandson. Upon his mother's departure from the room, this little boy would repeatedly throw out and reel back in a spool of thread whilst uttering words which both Freud and his daughter (Anna) interpreted as 'fort' and 'da', which, in German, mean 'gone' and 'there'. Freud speculated that the boy's behaviour indicated a repetition-compulsion, the psychological function of which was to adjust to the absence of the mother by enacting, in fantasy, the drama of her return. That is, the boy reassured himself that his mother and sole love-object would return by 'staging' that return in symbolic play, thereby mastering his anxieties through the use of his own imagination.

In many ways, this analysis of Freud's grandson contains all the basic elements of Klein's later approach. Before going on to look at that approach, however, we should pause to underline some important departures. Firstly, in both of these instances of Freud's own child analyses, he was actually interpreting accounts given by parents, not by children themselves. Nor, secondly, did he intervene therapeutically in their behaviour. Instead, he contented himself with a theoretical explanation that enlightened the concerned parents, but did not directly affect the child. Indeed, although Freud famously opened up to rigorous scrutiny the morphological twists and turns of infantile psycho-sexual development, he also based his insights, as I tried to show in chapter 4, on the retrospective constructions of *adult* patients. It was not children telling Freud about Oedipal desires as they experienced them, but adults recalling supposed childhood experiences from the vantage point of (a neurotically undermined) maturity. In stark contrast, Klein made enormous efforts to facilitate the child's own expression, and believed that she could make beneficial interventions into their emotional worlds by interpreting that expression. In so doing, she flouted the three basic tenets of classical Freudianism that had hitherto seemed to render the analysis of very young children impossible:

1. Children cannot recognise their neuroses *as* neuroses. Clearly, if neurotic symptoms are behaviours, emotions or thought processes that individuals experience as abnormal, it follows that these individuals must have some notion of normality by which to measure such deviations. But surely pre-Oedipal children have not yet been socialised into these wider norms? They know only how they feel, and not how these feelings correspond to the perceptions of others.
2. Given that children have comparatively under-developed linguistic skills, they are not in a position to take part in Freud's famous 'talking cure'. Without a profound understanding of language, the child cannot express its most complicated emotions. Yet from the earliest days of Freud and Breuer's 'cathartic method' with hysterics, the patient's therapeutic progress was reliant upon a verbalisation of repressed feelings and thoughts.
3. 'Transference' – whereby the patient is able to work through ambivalence towards important figures in their personal lives (typically parents) by projecting onto the analyst – is thought by classical Freudianism to be problematic in children because of their reluctance to identify with anything but parental figures. For young children, for whom parents and siblings constitute almost the entire emotional universe, identifying with adult strangers is naturally difficult, and this is no different with analysts.

So how did Klein challenge these assumptions at the core of classical Freudianism? Her principal insight was that children's play is a mode of communication (as Freud had already implied in relation to 'Little Hans') *but also* (as Freud had not stated) a site of potential therapeutic intervention. Specifically, Klein introduced the methodological innovation of treating children's play as *a non-verbal form of free-association*. A child's play, argued Klein, can be just as eloquent about unconscious fantasies as the verbalisations of an adult patient. The way children play, even in absolute silence, reveals aspects of their psychological state. Furthermore, play is a way of 'working through' anxieties resulting from these unconscious fantasies ('working through' indicates anything that facilitates the gradual acceptance of a potentially difficult psychological fact, such as mourning as a way of coming to terms with the death of a loved one). As one of Klein's ablest commentators puts it, '[i]n his play the child dramatizes his phantasies, and in doing so elaborates and works through his conflicts'.[1]

At first, Klein analysed children in their homes. However, she soon found that the presence of parents and siblings and the range of toys in the home were not conducive to genuinely expressive play. Instead, she invited her young patients to a separate and custom-designed room that was welcoming but neutral. She also restricted the range of available toys to objects that enabled the child to express its feelings about its relations with others. For example, she included toy houses that could symbolise home, and wooden figures which were identifiable as male or female, and which came in two different sizes, potentially indicating adults or other children. There were also farms and wild animals, as well as plasticine, scissors, string and pencils and paper. During analysis, Klein would simply encourage the children to play with these toys, watch them closely, and perhaps, after a couple of sessions, begin interacting with them as they played. Eventually, Klein would attempt to interpret, through a psychoanalytic framework, the symbolic meaning of these games and imagined scenarios. Using language that was simple, sensitive, and faithful to the unconscious world she had glimpsed, Klein would actually explain her interpretations to the child. It is this careful re-description of play that constitutes the therapeutic intervention in Kleinian child analysis. If these re-descriptions are accurate, the child will alter his or her play. Klein therefore measured her success by increases in the freedom and creative scope of the child's imaginative life. Sometimes, such changes were quite dramatic, since the children brought to her by worried parents were often insular and borderline autistic. These key elements of the Kleinian approach retain important aspects of the 'talking cure', insofar as a certain cathartic release is attained through the rendering conscious of unconscious material: by giving the children insight into the unconscious symbolism behind their own phantasies, the anxieties attached to them become dissipated.

Let us look at this in practice. One of Klein's early cases was a little boy called Peter, who, at age three, was already showing signs of psychological disturbance. He was nervous and clingy, easily frustrated, and deeply inhibited. During his sessions with Klein, an odd theme repeated itself in his play: he would violently knock together two wooden horses, and say 'I've got a little brother called Fritz'. Initially, the action and the words seemed unrelated. However, after Klein asked him what the horses were doing, Peter withdrew into his shell, stating 'that's not nice'. Just as Freud diagnosed resistance when a patient's free-associations dried up, so Klein intuited that Peter's game revealed his own fears and desires, and his inability to deal with them. At the next session, Klein decided to make a guess as to the symbolic meaning of the horses, by suggesting to Peter that the bumping horses were actually two people. Peter initially reacted with the

[1] Segal, Hanna. *Klein* (Glasgow: Fontana, 1979), p. 36.

same guarded expression: 'that's not nice'. However, his play then changed. He now laid the horses down flat, covered them in wooden bricks, and declared that they were quite dead! To the untrained ear, this perhaps sounds more disturbed and disturbing than ever, but Klein viewed this as a positive step forward. Why? Because Peter was enriching his own imaginative world, freeing up his own expression, and thereby turning play into an instrument for 'working through' his own anxieties. Subsequent sessions enabled Klein to flesh out this interpretation. Eventually, she felt she had determined that the root of Peter's problems lay in the anxiety he had been feeling since the arrival of his little brother (after his parents had 'bumped their thingummies together' like the toy horses). Again, she felt her speculations were therapeutically justified in the observable changes in Peter's behaviour, which became much more imaginative and creative.

So what did Klein discover through this form of play analysis with very young children, and how did it lead her to adapt classical Freudian psychoanalytic theory? One of the first things she discovered, as Peter's example demonstrates, is that parental figures are absolutely central to a child's fantasy life. Many games boiled down to the dramatisation of relations with mummy or daddy. At first glance, this sounds a very banal finding. Surely, such young children have few people in their lives *except* mummy and daddy. We shouldn't be surprised, then, that they crop up in their play. However, what Klein found was not that children simply mimicked scenarios previously experienced with their actual parents. Rather, their play expressed their emotional connections to the *psychic symbols* of parental figures. That is, 'real' external relations between the child and its parents were much less important than an internal – but, for the child, no less real – psychological relationship to parental symbols. Crucially, moreover, Klein found that children experienced deep-seated ambivalence in relation to these symbolic parental figures: sometimes they were caring and benevolent, but more often they were terrifying and malevolent.

In fact, Klein's findings indicated that 'the child, from the very beginnings of life, is consumed with anxiety and racked by destructive drives that put him in danger of being disintegrated'.[2] Gone is the image of an idyllic innocence and serenity of childhood, replaced by the notion that our very earliest years are strongly marked by aggression, frustration and self-persecutory anxiety. Immediately, and despite her fidelity to Freud, Klein's clinical discoveries challenged psychoanalytic orthodoxy. For Freud, as we have seen, the super-ego is formed only upon the resolution of the Oedipus Complex around the age of six. Prior to this period, claims Freud, the child cannot experience guilt or shame. Yet Klein disputed this chronology on the basis that her observation of children's play revealed powerful persecutory

[2] Kristeva, Julia. *Melanie Klein* (New York: Columbia University Press, 2001), p. 61.

forces at work long before the Oedipal phase. Indeed, this anxiety seemed to go back so far that these scary parental figures initially manifest themselves as 'part objects' because they precede the infant's awareness of its parents, particularly its mother, as a whole and separate entity. This fact necessitates a look at the importance of 'object relations theory' in Kleinian thought.

Object Relations

Generally, in psychoanalysis, the word 'object' means 'person'. However, it means 'person' not in reference to an actual person, but as they are experienced by a particular subject. Object relations theory therefore concentrates on the psychology of an individual's relations to their objects, or significant others, and the way these objects are set up and interrelate within their minds. It emphasises not how people interact (how does x get on with y), but rather the psychological value of the representation of a person, or 'object', in an individual's psychology (what does y *mean* to x). What object relations theory recognises is just how central to the human condition is the need for relations with others. To some extent, this position contradicts the orthodox 'instinct theory' posited by Freud, which argues that the main mechanism motivating behaviour is the regulation of instinctual tensions. This involves the libidinal energy attached to excess psychic excitation being 'siphoned' off by cathexis (as we saw in chapter 2, in relation to the pleasure principle). With object relations, this mechanical problem of regulating instinctual tension is secondary to an emphasis on the mind as a kind of internal theatrical stage peopled by various 'internal objects' which are the actors in the psychic dramas of fantasy.

Klein argued that the first such object was the mother's breast. For the suckling infant, it is the breast that supplies pleasure and to which it has an emotional relation of want and satisfaction. At this early stage, the breast is only a 'part object', because the baby is not yet aware of the mother as a being in her own right. Moreover, even at this early stage, the baby experiences ambivalence towards the part object of the breast. This is because the breast is a source of satisfaction on the one hand, insofar as it provides pleasure and nourishment, but on the other hand, it is also a source of frustration and anxiety, insofar as it seems unreliable. Sometimes the breast is there, but sometimes it is not: its presence or absence does not map onto the ebb and flow of the child's felt needs as seamlessly as it would like. Babies are so demanding largely because they have concepts neither of an outside world beyond their control, nor of the deferral of satisfaction that the separation between self and non-self necessitates. From the point of view of the grumpy little newborn, the pain of hunger is an inexplicable injustice. From the outset, the child both loves and hates the part object of the mother's breast which is the focus of this play of wants and their intermittent satisfaction as well as frustration. According to Klein, the aggression and anxiety induced by this situation, in which the child is utterly dependent on something that seems rather capricious and even cruel, threatens to overwhelm it.

Immediately, the child must develop defence mechanisms to fend off its own uncontrollable emotions, and perhaps the first of these is 'splitting'. By splitting the part object of the mother's breast into a good and a bad breast, the child is able to resolve its own ambivalence by separating the two contradictory feelings which it actually experiences simultaneously into two separate psychic symbols. The fiction of the wholly good breast that this enables, however, comes at quite a high cost. That cost is persecutory anxiety, for now the child is haunted by a terrifying bad breast which torments it, despite being nothing more than a reflection of its own innate frustration and aggression. Already, we can see the importance of the play between the introjection of objects (we have already seen this with Freud's account of the internalisation of the father figure at the Oedipal stage), and projection, which involves attributing merely mental and subjective phenomena to external agents. So here we have the little baby introjecting the breast as an internal part-object, splitting it into good and bad parts as a means of dealing with its own ambivalence, and then projecting that bad breast onto the actual breast.

According to Klein, babies that refuse to breast-feed may already be reacting to the bad breast that they have set up as an internal part-object: they experience the actual breast as evil and destructive. In contrast to Freud's model of subject formation, which emphasises the regulation of libidinal energy, Klein puts the introjection-projection relationship at the heart of the development of the ego. Much of Kleinian therapy, even with older patients, is therefore about setting up or reinforcing 'good' internal objects (these become whole objects as the child grows older, as we will see in a moment), and ensuring that these are projected outwards in a positive way which enhances personal interrelations.

The Paranoid-Schizoid Position

These insights into object relations allowed Klein, later in her career, to provide a detailed description of the very earliest defence mechanisms the child develops to cope with its innate ambivalence, which she called the 'paranoid-schizoid position'. It is a position, and not a stage in Freud's more deterministic terminology, because it is a configuration of object-relations that, while normally left behind as a part of ego-development, can nonetheless reappear at any time in life because of various external reasons. For example, a Kleinian interpretation of the behaviour of a schizophrenic would include the assumption that the schizoid coping strategies adopted in the first two years of life are resurfacing in the adult's manic behaviour.

By the time Klein was describing the paranoid-schizoid position, she was starting to take much more seriously than even the Freudians Freud's late notion of the death instinct, which we mentioned in passing in Chapter 5. Although the death instinct remained relatively vague in Freud's thought, Klein felt it described very well the innate aggression she had witnessed from her earliest analyses of children. With this new take on innate aggression, Klein believed that what the child must find defence mechanisms to cope with was actually its own self-destructive death instinct and the fundamental anxiety that came with it. The important point here is that all this anxiety and innate fear of death comes from within. For Kleinians, the fear of a destructive force coming from within is actually far more terrifying and primordial than the merely external threat of castration that Freud describes with the Oedipus Complex. Klein's paranoid-schizoid position describes the nascent ego's attempts to manage all this innate anxiety. She argues that it accomplishes this through five interrelated primitive defence mechanisms: splitting, as we have already seen, projection, introjection, idealisation and denial.

Splitting can occur at two different levels. Firstly, it can relate to the dividing of an object-representation into part-objects. This is what we have already seen with the good and bad breast. The paranoid part of the paranoid-schizoid position stems from the fear of attack from the projected bad breast (as with the baby that refuses to suckle, because the breast is experienced as malevolent). Idealisation refers to the flipside of this process, whereby the good object is set up as wholly good. This kind of idealisation, precisely because it is incongruous with reality, requires the compensation of denial: in order to continue with the illusion that someone or something is perfect, it is necessary to deny the evidence of their actual imperfection. This is what the little child does when it resolutely refuses to believe that the breast that gives it its most intense moments of pleasure is precisely the same breast that also causes it pain and hunger. After splitting, both denial and idealisation must combine to sustain the consoling illusion of an absolutely pure goodness and plenitude. The second way in which splitting can occur, however, is a splitting off of part of the ego itself. That is, aspects not of external objects, but of the young child's own personality and emotions, can be compartmentalised and separated. A version of this is present in Freud's idea of the super-ego, insofar as we experience the 'voice of our conscience' as if it were someone else's, an authority figure with strict moral values. However, while Freud explained this 'voice' as an introject of the father, Klein noticed that projection was also important.

Having split off unpleasant parts of its own ego, one of the main ways in which the child separates those parts is by projecting them outside of itself. Think of times when you have fallen out with friends. Very often, if we are honest, we would surely admit that we become angry with our friends not because of anything they have actually done, but because we are angry with *ourselves*, but in order to protect our own egos it is simply easier to blame someone else! Yet this very basic (and childish) defence mechanism has another dimension, according to Klein, and she called this 'projective identification'. This involves the split off component of the ego being projected outwards, but then, crucially, being *identified* with. Perhaps we can understand this with an example. Imagine a mugger. In order to keep stealing old ladies' handbags, he must somehow drown out the persecutory voice of his own moral conscience. He does this by splitting off that part of his ego, separating it from his sense of selfhood. However, one day, one of his victims fights back, and manages to detain him long enough to get him arrested. At his trial, the mugger projects his persecutory ego onto the magistrate who finds him guilty. In one of those logical irrationalities that we all use to justify our behaviour at times, our petty thief then blames the magistrate for his current predicament. In this way, he can behave as if it were the cruelty of this adjudicating individual, rather than the illegality of his own actions, that have led him to be stuck behind bars. This example illustrates how projective identification is a defence mechanism that separates components of the self: rather than addressing the difficult fact of his own immoral behaviour, the mugger projects his denied guilt and imagines himself a victim! Rather than channelling persecutory anxiety inwards towards his own ego, he directs it outwards, in the form of aggression towards the projection he is identifying with (the judge).

If in the adult this enables the avoidance of guilt, in the young child this pattern of projective identification can have serious consequences. The projection of bad objects can clearly lead to paranoia, or the feeling that 'the world is out to get me'. Yet even the projection of good objects can lead to loss of self-esteem on the one hand – since one is always going to suffer by comparison with an idealisation – or, on the other, severe disappointment and even despair, as one idealised object after another fails to live up to the perfection being ascribed to it. What Klein describes under the heading of the 'paranoid-schizoid' position is a perfectly normal stage of development which, as a rule, we pass through in the first year or so of life. Nonetheless, as a position, we can return to these same strategic defence-mechanisms at any time, and the pathological outcomes of adult recourse to the paranoid-schizoid position are particularly serious. The schizoid defence mechanisms of splitting, projection and denial can lead to a profoundly fragmented personality, for which symbolic meaning and a unified sense of self are beyond reach. Thus, the voices in the head of the schizophrenic pertain to the multiple split-off components of what used to be an ego, but which is now scattered and incoherent. In such a case, the self has been swamped by its own anxiety and its reliance on the primitive mechanism of splitting to try and cope with that anxiety.

The Depressive Position

The position that, in the normal course of development, succeeds the paranoid-schiziod position, is called by Klein the 'depressive position'. This is more 'mature' than the paranoid-schizoid position insofar as it involves the recognition of whole objects as opposed to part-objects: the 'breast-object' starts to become the 'mummy-object'. Because of improved perception and memory, the child can recall the satisfaction the mother provided for him even when she is not physically present (he can therefore start to trust in her return). This in turn allows a reduction in the strategy of splitting, so that the child can face the previously inadmissable fact that the good and bad breast are one and the same thing. With this relative abandonment of schizoid splitting, a comparative integration of the child's ego becomes possible. However, this recognition of other whole objects is not yet accompanied by a robust sense of the separation between an inside and an outside, between the child's mind, and external reality. Indeed, the fundamental trait of the depressive position is that this indeterminacy between inside and outside becomes the source of profound anxiety because the child cannot differentiate between the violence of its own fantasies, and the independent continuity of the whole objects around it, particularly 'mummy'.

At the heart of the depressive position then, is a play between innate aggression and the anxiety attending the perceived consequences of that aggression. This is because, as we have already seen, introjection is one of the most important ways for the nascent ego to establish itself. The child, having split the breast into good and bad objects, tries to externalise the bad breast (which is a representation of the child's own death drive), but it also tries to introject the good breast, to bring the good breast into its own emotional world as a constant and reassuring presence (this is how the ego fortifies itself). The same strategy is applied to the whole object of the mother when she starts to be experienced as more than just a breast. Unfortunately, once ensconced in this internal psychic reality, the introjected whole object of the mother is completely exposed in the child's fantasy life to all its sadistic tendencies. Now, even the utterly good internal mother can be (psychically) destroyed by the aggressive impulses of the death drive! Because the child does not yet have a sense of separation between its own fantasies and external reality, a new set of emotions become possible at this point: loss, sorrow, pining, but also guilt. In the same proportion that the good object was the embodiment of perfection and ultimate satisfaction, so its absence, after the fantasy of its destruction, becomes a deep well of sadness and remorse for the child. This is why Klein calls this configuration the depressive position, although it does not *yet* have direct connections with clinical depression *per se* (we will see what the actual connection is in a moment).

This cataclysmic psychological event leads to acute anxiety, to the extent that the child suddenly feels that all its internal good objects are both ambiguous and frighteningly fragile. For this reason, it is of paramount importance during the depressive position that the actual mother is around the child in a consistent and reliable way. Only by demonstrating the continuity of her love, in spite of the destructive fantasies to which she is subjected in the child's internal world, can the child be persuaded of the distinction between her external reality and her psychic representation. Put simply, even if in his play the child finds himself smashing symbols of his mother to pieces and then feeling dreadful guilt, eventually, the fact that mother herself keeps coming to him and giving him reassurance and comfort anyway, establishes for him both the difference between fantasy and reality, and the notion of a less precarious good object who will always be there for him.

These insights of Klein's align with an important aspect of today's child psychology, called 'Attachment Theory', proposed primarily by John Bowlby. Attachment Theory emphasises the importance of parental love in endowing the child with a sense that those they invest in emotionally will be reliable, and that they themselves are worthy of love. Although not a psychoanalytic theory, Bowlby's claim about the impact of secure or insecure parental bonds on future relationships matches well with Klein's claims about the damage that can be done if the inconsistency of the mother in particular allows the child to continue imagining that his fantasy life is imposed on outer reality.

For Klein, imperfect emergence from the depressive position can lead to irrational guilt. For example, in later life, such a person might react to the death of a loved one by blaming themselves, as if they were personally responsible. This can lead to what Freud called melancholia, which is an arrested kind of mourning. It is for this reason that much Kleinian analysis of adults concentrates on what she calls 'reparation', which simply means making good the damage the patient imagines they have done, in phantasy,[3] to the internal good object, re-creating it anew if necessary.

[3] Charles Rycroft points out that English psychoanalysts influenced by Klein use this particular spelling to indicate the underlying power of imagination behind all mental activity, as opposed to the 'caprice, whim, fanciful invention' that defines 'fantasy' in common usage. See Rycroft, Charles, *A Critical Dictionary of Psychoanalysis* (London: Penguin, 1995), pp. 55-56.

8 Lacan: the Split Subject

Despite being probably the most esoteric and impenetrable theorist imaginable, the French psychoanalyst Jacques Lacan (1901-1981) has also had probably the greatest intellectual impact of any analyst since Freud. His ideas have touched, even transformed, various disciplines, from continental philosophy to Film Studies, literary theory to analyses of consumer culture. In part, we can explain the apparent contradiction between his difficulty and his broad impact in terms of the diversity of bodies of thought upon which he draws. In the dauntingly difficult tapestry of his texts, there are woven threads from Marxism, Existentialism, Hegelianism, Phenomenology, Anthropology, Saussurean linguistics, and even Surrealism! In part, too, we should explain Lacan's appeal in terms of the abiding attraction of his description of the human condition, which renders our existence highly dramatic, dynamic, and yet, somehow, also irretrievably doomed. The 'split subject' which Lacan describes is a deeply tragic character, as we will see.

Lacan is also an exemplary 'post-Freudian' in the sense we have been using here, because although he famously advocated 'a return to Freud', his ideas are extremely resistant to being assimilated to any of the main branches of psychoanalysis. This was reflected in his personal biography. Despite becoming something of a cult hero in post-war French intellectual life, he resigned from the *Société Psychoanalytique de Paris* in 1953, and allowed his membership of the International Psychoanalytic Association to lapse completely in that same year. This meant that his most influential ideas were formulated very much on the peripheries of institutionalised forms of psychoanalysis, where he was regarded by many as something of an intellectual charlatan. Lacan can therefore be viewed with some justification as the *enfant terrible* of psychoanalytic theory. It is certainly true that, despite his professed fidelity to Freud, he took the movement in directions that its originator could not have even dreamed of. Indeed, to enter Lacan's densely philosophical world is to plunge headlong into a radical critique of the idea of the subject put forward by the philosopher Descartes, an idea which seemed to influence even Freud's model of the mind, but which with Lacan becomes a mere side-effect of language.

In order at least to loosen, if not untie, the Gordian (or Borromean?) knot that is Lacanian theory, we will concentrate on two seminal essays before expanding on the interrelations between his three key terms, the Imaginary, the Symbolic and the Real. This approach has the unfortunate effect of presenting a version of Lacan relevant primarily to his earliest writings, repressing a 'later Lacan' who makes rather different emphases (particularly around the idea of the 'real'). To redress this imbalance, the committed reader is directed to Bruce Fink's *The Lacanian Subject.*[1]

[1] Fink, Bruce. *The Lacanian Subject: Between Language and Jouissance* (Princeton: Princeton University Press, 1995).

The Mirror Stage

In some ways, Lacan's 1949 essay, 'The Mirror-Stage as Formative of the Function of the I as Revealed in Psychoanalytic Experience',[2] deals with many of the issues we have seen Melanie Klein wrestling with. It too focuses on the earliest months of the infant's life and it too is centrally concerned with the development of the sense of selfhood. Moreover, it too qualifies Freud's narrative of the Oedipal stage. However, whereas Klein emphasised the play of introjection and projection in the delineation of the ego's boundaries, Lacan stresses the role of the image in establishing an apparent unity of the self.

Lacan argues that, unlike most animals in the natural world, human beings are effectively born prematurely, so that in the first months of life, the infant is 'still trapped in his motor impotence and nursling dependence'.[3] As if not quite prepared for the world, infants before the age of six months are a mere aggregate of disconnected drives, impulses and primitive stimuli responses. Because of this incoherent form of existence, they cannot differentiate themselves from their surroundings. For Lacan, the interesting question becomes: if we start life as disorganised bundles of drives and sensations without unity, how, out of this confusing morass, does a coherent sense of self emerge? What is the trigger for the transition from being a mere body to becoming a 'subject' with a sense of identity? Lacan tries to answer this question by evoking a primordial scene: that of the infant before the mirror.

It is only in front of the mirror, claims Lacan, that the child can become aware of its own body as a totality with specific borders. At first, the infant before its reflection may experience its own image simply as if it were a separate reality, another 'thing' to engage with. This is a stage before even that of the domestic cat which, in front of its own reflection, will arch its back, hiss, and launch a vicious attack on its own likeness *as if it were another cat*. This aggressively territorial reaction is of course based on an albeit mistaken recognition: the cat assumes it is faced by another cat. The infant, however, is still unaware of itself as a 'self', and therefore does not recognise the image in the looking glass as even another baby, let alone as its own likeness.

However, if the infant is allowed to spend enough time before the mirror, it will start to conceive of a relationship between the virtual complex of polymorphous sensations which is, at this stage, its only mode of awareness, and corresponding changes in the image. That is to say, the sensation of even an involuntary motion of an arm will correspond to a resultant motion in the image. By watching this correspondence and experimenting with it, the infant discovers, in its reflection, an image of its own unity. This

[2] Lacan, Jacques. *Écrits*, trans. Bruce Fink (London: Norton, 2006), pp. 75-81

[3] Lacan, *Écrits*, p. 76.

becomes the origin of the infant's sense of self, as a kind of container which gathers the diffuse and polymorphous bundle of drives and sensations which it had hitherto been. For Lacan, this is a crucial pre-requisite for Freud's Oedipal Complex. Freud's Oedipal narrative emphasises the emergence of the ego from socialising forces, but Lacan invokes a pre-social, rather more existential ego which must already be in place for the Oedipal phase to get under way, and thus for the social 'I' to emerge.

> [The mirror-stage] would seem to exhibit in an exemplary situation the symbolic matrix in which the *I* is precipitated in a primordial form, before it is objectified in the dialectic of identification with the other, and before language restores to it, in the universal, its function as subject.[4]

Like Klein, Lacan stresses the importance of the earliest months of pre-Oedipal life but, unlike Klein, he places great importance on the visual, and on the gaze. To support this power of visuality in identity formation, he cites the fact that pigeons, in order to develop fully functioning reproductive organs, must *see* other pigeons, of either sex (and this can be induced by using mirrors). Similarly, locusts can convert to a 'gregarious' form suitable to life in a swarm simply by *seeing* other locusts.[5] In a related way, the human infant can become a coherent *I* only by seeing itself in the mirror.

This all sounds entirely plausible, and one is tempted to move on a little too quickly by simply accepting that a unified self has now been constructed with the help of the mirror image. However, with Lacan, things are never so simple. For, in fact, this moment of the infant's identification with its reflection, even as it makes the pre-Oedipal 'I' possible, is also, paradoxically, the moment that makes *complete* unity and *complete* identity simultaneously impossible! Here, we come upon the first split in the Lacanian split subject. The infant, as it becomes a self, is also split from itself because what it identifies with – its reflection – is *only* an image. Very obviously, one's reflection is not oneself, but something exterior, separate, necessarily always different from one's interior life. Nonetheless, an indispensable part of the mirror-stage is experiencing and accepting the mirror image *as* reality, and moreover, as the reality of one's self. Lacan calls this process of the experience of a mere image as a reality *méconnaissance*, which simply means 'misrecognition' (but also, in French, has an important resonance with 'mis-knowledge'). To recognise for the first time the possibility of its unified totality, the infant must *mis*recognise its reflection *as* itself. This originating split is therefore between our bodily, unmediated experience of biological life on the one hand, and on the other an external image of unity that forever separates us from ourselves but

[4] Lacan, *Écrits*, p. 2.
[5] Lacan, *Écrits*, p. 3.

which also makes any sense of self possible in the first place.

Indeed, it is in view of *méconnaissance* that Lacan introduced into psychoanalysis the term 'alienation', which he took, greatly modified, from Marxism. Early Marx complained that factory workers during the period of industrialisation were 'alienated' from their own work. The products that they made with their own hands had no direct meaning in their lives (often they could not afford to purchase these products themselves). In fact, such workers became mere extensions of the machinery of mass production. For Marx, this meant that man becomes alienated from his own 'species-being' as labour is less and less integrated with the organic needs of a community. Lacan takes this idea, which is really social rather than psychological, and radicalises it. Whereas in Marx this alienation was seen as the outcome of a specific mode of production called Capitalism (which would be surpassed by Communism), Lacan removes this historical contingency by making *the subject in general constitutively alienated from itself.* According to Lacan, the subject only emerges in and through the double-bind of the mirror-stage, which demands an identification with something resolutely separate from the self, a mere image or *imago*. This makes alienation and misrecognition a condition of all subjectivity: we will always be searching for our true identities outside of ourselves.

Thus, in Lacan's rather bleak theoretical world, our sense of self is always a trap, a lure and a deception. Identity takes on a paranoiac structure, insofar as the only way we can unify the fragmented body that we were as infants – and that, beneath the illusory totality of the 'self', we still are as adults – is to find validation in others. We stare anxiously into the eyes of others to see if we can see ourselves reflected there. In fact, Lacan claims that what we really come to desire is the desire of the Other. Yet the Other cannot provide us with the unconditional affirmation we crave, since the gap between self and image, thing and representation, creates a hole at the centre of our being.

This hole can never be filled, yet much of our emotional life represents an endless quest for the illusory wholeness we first saw in the mirror. Later in his career, Lacan argued that we go through life seeking what he called the 'object a', through which we attempt to recover the pleasure (Lacan calls this '*jouissance*') associated with our early unity with the mother. The 'object a' explains why we move so restlessly from one source of external validation to another, whether sporting achievement, academic excellence, sexual adventure, or even drug addiction. It is also the very motor of our fantasy life, insofar as we construct fantasies that satisfy, in a hallucinatory form, our desire finally to find 'object a' in the form of an ultimate sexual union, sublime wealth, celebrity or popularity. Yet ultimately, none of these things will truly satisfy us: contentment, like the horizon, recedes as we approach it. Although a predictable component of social life, this search for stable and meaningful self-integrity through others – and, in a consumer society, increasingly through 'things' – is also, for Lacan, unfaithful to the dynamic reality of psychic life. Malcolm Bowie puts this well:

> [T]he 'alienating destination' of the 'I' is such that the individual is permanently in discord with himself: the 'I' is tirelessly intent upon freezing a subjective process that cannot be frozen, introducing stagnation into the mobile field of human desire.[6]

As we will see later, these two elements – self-alienation through the misrecognition of the image, and the (vain) search for something external with which to fill the lack at the core of being – are brought together by Lacan under the heading of the Imaginary.

The Agency of the Letter

If the mirror-stage essay is the founding statement of Lacan's rather dark, existentialist view of the incompletable subject, his other famous essay, 'The Agency of the Letter in the Unconscious, or Reason since Freud,'[7] represents his most radical revision of the Freudian unconscious. Much of this essay's radicalism comes from the unprecedented centrality it gives to language, and to the constitution of the subject *through* language at a stage which follows the mirror-stage. Although Lacan claimed that language had always been at the forefront of Freud's theories and clinical practice, citing Freud's close analyses of jokes, parapraxes, and dreams, it was Lacan who brought to psychoanalysis the rigour of modern linguistics, and thus a set of conceptual tools that largely post-dated Freud.

To understand Lacan's difficult ideas in this essay, we must start by outlining in some detail the key tenets put forward by the revolutionary Swiss linguist, Ferdinand de Saussure, who can be considered the father of modern linguistics, and of whose ideas Lacan makes idiosyncratic use in 'The Agency of the Letter'.

Saussurean Linguistics

We can grasp Saussure's approach to language by expanding on two of his most important claims, namely 'the relationality of meaning' and 'the arbitrariness of the sign'. The first claim immediately flies in the face of

[6] Bowie, Malcolm. *Lacan* (London: Fontana, 1991), p. 25.
[7] See Lacan, *Écrits*, pp.146-178.

how we tend to think of language. After all, in the normal course of things we assume that words act rather like labels for things that they serve to designate. The word 'dog' for example, designates four-legged furry creatures that show the characteristics of the genus 'canine'. What could be simpler than the idea that the actual dog is the referent of the word 'dog'? However, Saussure, in his famous (although posthumous) *Course in General Lingustics* argued that in order to function, the label must always have a relationship with other labels. Indeed, there is a whole system for arranging the differences between such labels which is not apparent in individual utterances, but upon which every act of speech is nonetheless entirely dependent if it is to be meaningful.

Thus, part of the meaning of the word 'dog' derives from its negative relation to other words: 'dog' functions in the way it does, not because it has some essential relation to its referent (the furry four-legged creature), but because it is not 'log' or 'dot' or 'dig', and so on. It is the relation between other sounds and concepts that allows any given utterance to convey a meaning. To understand how meaning comes about, one must examine the function of a given utterance within this larger system of differences. Every statement effectively invokes the whole of this larger structure, although it remains implicit rather than explicit. Thus, while most linguists before Saussure were philologists and etymologists who concentrated on the evolution of languages and how it impacted on current usage, Saussure emphasised *formal* structure in the here and now. He therefore examined a system, rather than a history, of meaning.

Saussure made two distinctions that helped circumscribe the proper object of study for modern linguistics. Firstly, he opposed a 'synchronic' to a 'diachronic' approach. The former was his preferred formal and structural analysis of language at a specific moment in time, while the latter was that approach which stressed the changing history of a language *over* time. Secondly, he opposed what he called *langue* (language) to *parole* (speech). *Parole* designated the plane of the actual utterance, of the specific linguistic act, but what Saussure was really concerned with was the formal structure which made that act possible, and it was this that he called *langue*. This was a major change in the way language had been conceived, and because of its emphasis on structure, it became known as 'structural linguistics'. This in turn gave birth to a vibrant and wide-ranging intellectual movement that was particularly important in post-war French thought, called Structuralism, which impacted on everything from poetics to anthropology, and which provided the intellectual milieu in which Lacan was to write his essay on the unconscious.

A fundamental outcome of Saussure's emphasis on the relationality of meaning was the concomitant recognition of what he called the arbitrariness of the sign. That is to say, Saussure demonstrated that there is no ontological or even onomatopoeic connection between a word or concept and its referent. Put simply, there is nothing dog-like about the word 'dog'. Because meaning, or what Structuralists prefer to call 'signification', emerges from a system of differences (*langue*), we could just as well designate that four-legged furry canine creature with 'cat', 'kettle' or 'carburettor'! It is only our conventional familiarity with the existing *langue* that makes such a proposition seem so absurd. So although words (or signs) seem far from arbitrary to us, they *are* arbitrary on the level of *langue*, where there is no need for a positive relation of correspondence (no need, that is, for the word dog somehow to resemble actual dogs), but only a negative relation of difference

Perhaps we can make this difficult point more forcefully by looking at two paintings by the Belgian Surrealist, René Magritte, who definitely understood Saussure's point. (We are not even straying far from psychoanalysis here, as of all artistic movements of the twentieth century, Surrealism was certainly the one most influenced by Freud's ideas, and in Magritte we have a painter-philosopher who was clearly fascinated by language too.)

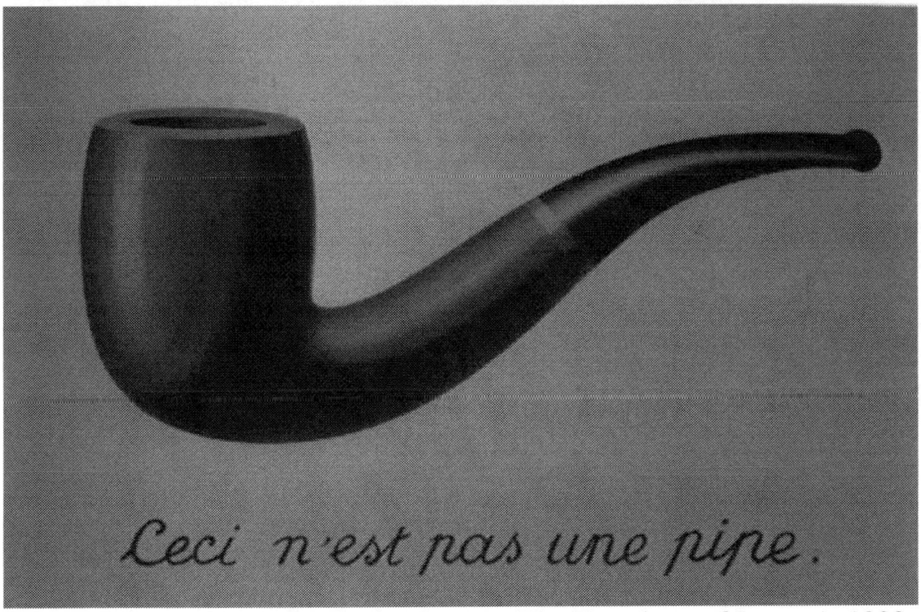

Magritte, René, *La Trahison des Images* (The Treachery of Images), 1929. Oil on canvas, 25 x 37 inches.
Collection: Los Angeles County Museum of Art.

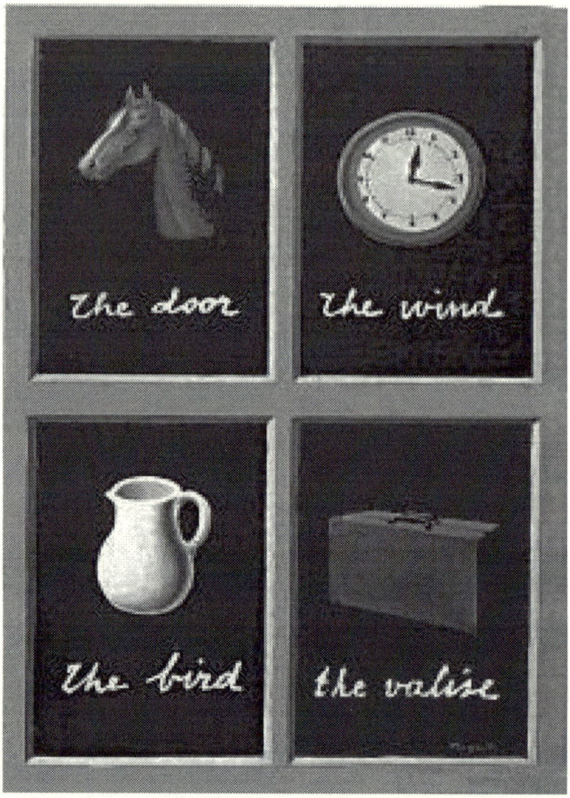

Magritte, René, *Le clef des songes* (The Key of Dreams), 1935.
Oil on canvas, 16 x 10 ½ inches.
Collection: Jasper Johns.

The first painting reinforces well the very point that Lacan was making in his essay on the mirror-stage. Even though the image is a realistic representation of a pipe, and even though, if asked, we would surely declare that it was indeed a pipe, there is nonetheless nothing here into which one could stuff tobacco and light! Magritte is illustrating the same gap between representation and thing that Lacan had explored in relation to the mirror-image and the sense of self. Saussure's terminology helps us to describe this gap, because he makes an important distinction between what he calls the 'signifier' and the 'signified'. Here is a quick Saussurean glossary:

Signifier: the thing carrying the meaning (this could be a sound, an image, an object, a gesture or even a smell, but it always has a material dimension).

1. Signified: the concept that is conveyed (what we commonly refer to as the 'meaning').

2. Sign: the combination of the signifier and signified (Saussure says that it is only in the abstract that these can be separated anyway).

To use these terms in relation to Magritte's first painting, we can say that the signifier here is simply oil paint on canvas. Now, normally, we would say that, thanks to the conventions of realism, the signified conveyed is simply 'pipe'. However, the text that Magritte introduces *into* the painting, 'this is not a pipe', complicates this signified. The higher-level signified then becomes an actual separation between signifier and signified which the sign normally covers over. It is in this sense that the 'treason of images' to which the title of this painting refers is homologous with the betrayal of the alienating image of the self in Lacan's mirror.

However, in the second painting – whose very title leads us to assume that Magritte was versed in Freudian dream-theory – great play is made of the arbitrariness of the sign. Here we have representations of objects to which are appended nouns that, with one exception, do not fit the visual representations. Thus, a horse becomes a 'door', a clock becomes 'the wind', and a jug becomes a 'bird'. Only the valise retains its conventional label. The fact that Magritte paints these objects in the manner of an infant's text book, of the 'A is for Apple' variety, suggests the merely learnt, or inherited, nature of the linguistic conventions that make these juxtapositions seem completely 'surreal'. Yet if one accepts Saussure's account of language, the image is actually a realistic account of how meaning works. So, if the first painting separates the signifier from the signified, this second painting illustrates the counter-intuitive arbitrariness of the sign as a whole, which allows any word to stand for any thing.

It is these two insights from Saussurean linguistics – the relationality of meaning and the arbitrariness of the sign – that Lacan brings to bear on the Freudian unconscious in his famous essay.

The Unconscious Structured Like a Language

We can now finally turn to Lacan's essay on the unconscious. However, even though Lacan makes use of these Saussurean ideas in his essay, it is important to note at the outset that he also radicalises them. According to Saussure, the signifier and the signified are sides of the same coin, and both are united in the stable 'sign'. There is no contamination of one by the other: the signifier simply supports the signified it is called upon to convey. The system of differences described by Saussure under the heading of *langue* is therefore rather static.

In contrast, Lacan claims that not only is the signified reliant upon its signifier instead of the other way around (already rather scandalous), but there is an incessant sliding of the signified under the signifier. We must be careful here, for it sounds as if Lacan might be saying that there is no such thing as a signified, only signifiers! However, this is not at all the case. Rather, he is arguing that the signifier is no longer a merely neutral or transparent vehicle for signification, and that the signified *needs* the signifier but cannot fully control it. If this is true, meaning immediately becomes slippery, dynamic and unstable, but this does not mean it does not take place. Indeed, it would be more accurate to say that meaning takes place in abundance, and in ways that cannot be regulated by the intervention of the 'intentional' speaking subject (this should already make us think of the unconscious even as Freud described it, as something antithetical to conscious intention).

So while Lacan's radicalisation of Saussure does suggest that signs are never really discrete units that support a fixed referent, he absolutely does not say that meaning is impossible (this would obviously be a self-contradictory statement). Rather, what meaning signs do possess is made possible only by their reliance on unruly signifiers and by their position within a chain of other signs. The signified is really a kind of pause, or ephemeral anchoring, in an otherwise ceaseless flux along that chain: 'we can say that it is in the chain of the signifier that meaning *insists*, but that none of the chain's elements *consists* in the signification it can provide at that very moment'.[8] Lacan uses the concept-metaphor of '*points de capiton*', which in French means upholstery or quilting button, to describe this anchoring of the sliding signifier. Like the button that gathers in and pins down upholstery fabric, the signified gathers in and pins down the elusive signifier to create a relatively stable meaning. Yet the text(ile) of signification will not be pinned down for long, and every signified must become the signifier of another sign, and so on *ad infinitum*.

If this all sounds rather complicated (and it surely does), perhaps we can simplify Lacan's point by summarising his idea of the 'slipperiness of the signifier' with a word we are more used to: 'poetry'. After all, we use the word 'poetry' to describe that aspect of language which is pregnant with elusive meaning. Poetry conveys things which prose cannot, exactly because it uses words and concepts in unconventional ways that nonetheless still create an affect or feeling in the reader. How would this be possible if all words functioned like precise labels, meaning exactly and always the same thing in all contexts? By stressing the role of the signifier, Lacan also stresses the poetic aspects of language, crucially, of *all* language and not just ostensibly literary expression. For example, a clear statement of fact can be transformed into its opposite simply by a sarcastic intonation. An order can cease to be an order when it is uttered in the context of a play at the theatre. Or, again, a statement can become 'contaminated' by an unintended double meaning. So if I say 'I wanted to stand at the top of Mount Everest

[8] Lacan, *Écrits*, p. 419.

for ten years', I could mean a) I have yearned for ten whole years to reach the top of that mountain, or b) once there, I intended to stay there for a whole decade (in rhetorical theory, this is called an amphiboly). These brief examples show how poetic or rhetorical aspects of language, such as intonation, context, and syntactical ambiguity, which are all connected to the material level of the signifier, have an important impact on the signified.

Having profoundly re-described the Saussurean landscape as inescapably 'poetic', Lacan goes on to apply this logic of the signifier to the Freudian unconscious. His fundamental claim is that psychoanalysis needs to purge itself of its residual biologism by ceasing to think of the unconscious as the seat of instinctual drives. Thus, it must replace that old dynamic model with the linguistic model just described, which, he claims, Freud was always concerned with anyway (whether he knew it or not). With Lacan, the unconscious has no existence outside or before speech. It is not some kind of archaic silence at the depths of our psyche that needs to be expressed in consciousness, but an ambiguity inherent to the speech through which we 'speak ourselves', or rather, through which we are spoken. Thus, Lacan argues that the distortions of the dream-work, for example, can be redescribed in terms of the 'agency of the letter', which is to say, in terms of the slippery or poetic properties of the signifier. No longer is the distortion of the dream-work to be understood as the modification of instinctual energy, but rather, as a direct effect of symbolic language, though an effect which does not coincide with consciousness. Thus, onto Freud's notions of displacement and condensation, Lacan maps the rhetorical terms 'metonymy' and 'metaphor', with metonymy describing the horizontal contiguity of signs (with parts standing in for the whole) and metaphor describing the vertical substitution of signs one for another. Here, Lacan is indebted to the linguist Roman Jakobson, who argued that all language functions along two axes, the syntagmatic and the paradigmatic. Yet as a psychoanalyst, Lacan is specifically concerned with the interrelations between language and subjectivity – that is, he is still interested in how we come to have a sense of self.

After all, these rather dry observations about language only take on their fullest *psychoanalytic* implications when one adopts Lacan's position, that *the 'I' is itself only a signifier*. This means that identity itself is completely wrapped up in the slippings and slidings of the Saussurean sign, and is not at all about a repressed essence striving for expression. For Lacan, the idea that there are people first, and then there is language, and people simply use language as a tool to give form to their inner reality, is a harmful illusion. On the contrary, identity is obtained in and through language and the one is implicated in the other. We are thrown, as it were, into this pre-existing structure or *langue* and through it we are constructed as subjects with a sense of self. Yet this sense of self is no more and no less than a mere signifier, prey to the incessant flux of signification.

Here we have the second split in the Lacanian split subject. If the first split related to the mirror-stage and the false (or imaginary) image of a unity of the self, this subsequent split relates to the insertion of our identities into the symbolic maelstrom of a shared language which never truly belongs to us. This has strange consequences for the way we tend to think of ourselves. In our narcissism, we tend to assume that our consciousness is *ours*, that we are unique in some way, that we are individuals whose personal histories, if nothing else, make us special. Yet Lacan's recourse to structural linguistics suggests that little of what we experience as uniquely 'ours' actually is.

It is also here that Lacan's major critique of the Cartesian subject can be discerned. Descartes was the philosopher who used a process of systematic doubt in order to come upon the seemingly irrefutable dictum of self-identity: *ego cogito ergo sum*, or 'I think therefore I am'. Lacan disagrees with this formulation because it rests on the notion that signifier and signified, here 'thinking' and 'being', are one and the same thing. To use Saussure's language, Descartes argues that we are ourselves in the form of a sign that completely reconciles signified and signifier. In fact, Lacan, somewhat echoing Magritte's painting of the pipe, says that there are really two types of subject here. One is the subject (in a grammatical, *and*, now, a psychoanalytic sense) of the signifier (here, the first 'I'), and one is the subject of the signified (the second 'I'). That is, when I speak of myself, I am trying to be the subject of the signifier 'I', but in labelling myself in this way, 'I' also become the referent or signified (see task 8 below). Later in his career, Lacan would make it clear that there is an important difference between the embodied individual and the subject, with the latter being a symbolic and interpersonal construct operated through language.

These are very difficult ideas, but perhaps it helps to keep in mind who Lacan was really targeting with this philosophical assault on the Cartesian cogito. His real target was the practitioners of what he felt to be a pernicious and largely American form of ego-psychology which concentrated on strengthening the ego *against* the unconscious. In Lacan's contrary view, the ego is actually the 'bad guy' in the psychic drama, insofar as it tries to freeze the flow of signification through various defence mechanisms which can lead to pathological outcomes. More often than not, observed Lacan in his clinical practice, the ego is *too* strong rather than not strong enough. As Bruce Fink puts it, "[t]he ego is so strong and rigid that repression occurs whenever one of the neurotic's own sexual or aggressive impulses does not fit in with his view of himself. There would be no symptoms were the neurotic's ego too weak to push such impulses outside of itself".[9] This shows that the Freud that Lacan called for a return to was really the early

[9] Fink, Bruce. *A Clinical Introduction to Lacanian Psychoanalysis: Theory and Technique* (London: Harvard University Press, 1997), p. 3.

Freud, and that Lacan never really accepted the id-ego-superego distinction. Thus, much of Lacan's recourse to the Saussurean notion of *langue*, as a pre-existing and deeply non-human technology of signification, must be conceived of in this context of a deliberate polemic against ego-psychology and its philosophical underpinnings in the Cartesian subject.

The Imaginary, the Symbolic and the Real

Now that we have unpacked some of Lacan's most dense ideas, we can quickly outline three of his most important terms. For Lacan's mature theory begins to articulate the two moments of splitting in the subject that we have examined in terms of three orders: the Imaginary, the Symbolic and the Real. Rather as Klein distances herself from Freud's determinism with her notion of 'positions', so Lacan insists on this notion of 'orders', rather than stages, because he wants to stress that each of his three key terms are co-implicated. Even though Lacan often presents his ideas in a narrative form, with the drama of the mirror-stage and the event of entry into language, the Imaginary, Symbolic and Real are nonetheless orders that serve to position the individual at different times and in different psychic-social spaces.

The Imaginary We have already seen the primary characteristics of the Imaginary in our account of the mirror-stage. The imaginary pertains to the image of plenitude in the mirror, the play of (self-)identification, and the perpetual demand for reciprocated love from the other. For Lacan, it is essentially a negative term, insofar as it describes a fairly desperate scene in which the individual is encouraged by the illusion of wholeness first glimpsed in the mirror to attempt, but always to fail, to fix identity. The ego is *the* Imaginary object, not in the sense that it does not exist, but in the sense that it is an illusory creation whose purpose is to resist the effects of the unconscious (through denial and rationalisation). The ego is therefore a sort of neurotic refusal of the flux of becoming, and it is the focus of Lacanian analysis. This refusal tends to come in the form of fantasies that hold out the promise of completion (in consumer culture, for example, the fantasy that buying a certain product will make you blissfully happy). However, as we have seen, such fantasies can only paper over the lack that is always at the core of selfhood. The ego itself is characterised by this doomed fantasy of unity, and much of Lacanian analysis therefore attempts to bypass the defences of the ego in order to 'subjectify' the Real around which the ego continually circles in a neurotic fashion. It is in this sense that Lacanian analysis is the antithesis of ego-psychology.

The Symbolic Again, we have already laid the ground-work for understanding the Symbolic order with our close attention to the essay on the 'Agency of the Letter'. For the Symbolic relates to language in Saussure's expanded sense of a system of differences, though now given added dynamism by Lacan's stress on the signifier. In contrast to the Imaginary, the Symbolic is generally a positive term in Lacan's usage, because it enables the kind of experimentation and creativity that Lacan approves of. It is also the realm of intersubjective communication and the inauguration of social bonds. Entering the Symbolic order is for Lacan the precondition for having existence at all, because it is only as a name or place-holder within the system of differences that one can be the subject of (one's own) discourse. As always with Lacan, however, the Symbolic has another side, which is that of the articulation of a perpetual desire. Lacan's notion of desire is very different from Freud's residually biological version, which conceived of a kind of reservoir of libido which the individual invests in various objects through cathexis. The Lacanian subject, in contrast, is at the mercy of his or her desire and cannot fully control its expression. Rather than a pre-existing libidinal reservoir, Lacanian desire is fundamentally intersubjective. It is the remainder that is left after you subtract need from demand, i.e., the fundamental 'hunger' that persists *after* the child has been fed, and its merely biological requirements have been met. Because of the lack at the heart of identity, the subject desires an unconditional and complete 'yes' from the Other that language enables (this Other is not the same as empirical others). Entry into the Symbolic therefore enables communication, so that, for example, the infant can cry out the word 'mummy' to express its state of need, yet the Symbolic also represents entry into a discourse of insatiable desire. On the cusp of the Symbolic then, the subject-to-be is faced with a dilemma: to be granted existence in language at all, one must renounce a pre-Oedipal *jouissance*[10] which has being, but does not exist (Lacan says it only 'ex-sists', which means it has a reality but one that language cannot testify to). Once the subject has taken the plunge into the Symbolic, they are left with an impoverished version of their original *jouissance*, which is the phallic *jouissance* enabled within language in the form of fantasy.

The Real The 'Real' is perhaps Lacan's most enigmatic concept, partly because the word itself is misleading. The Real is certainly not substitutable for any simplistic notion of 'reality'. Indeed, 'reality' is a construct of the socialised ego and is not therefore the level at which

[10] The French word *jouissance* means pleasure, but specifically a pleasure that also verges upon pain. It can also refer to orgasm. In early Lacan, it is what gets foreclosed from the Symbolic by castration, but in later Lacan, a certain *jouissance* comes to suffuse both language and knowledge and to take on a feminine, which is to say, a non-phallic character.

Lacanian analysis operates. Lacan's 'Real' is also in contrast with Freud's use of 'reality'. Freud tended to think of 'reality' as an empirical realm outside the subject, to the constraints of which the ego must adapt by imposing upon itself the 'reality principle'. Lacan, on the other hand, thinks of the Real as that which is entirely and irretrievably beyond the reach of the signifying chain. The Real can never be represented within the Symbolic. Indeed, Lacan makes the exclusion of the Real a structural condition of subjectivity in general, so that entry into the Symbolic is, once again, a kind of Faustian bargain which means renouncing the Real. Yet the loss of the Real is somehow felt, for example, as the loss of *jouissance* which, perhaps as a retrospective fantasy, we imagine we enjoyed with the mother. Thus, compensation for this loss of *jouissance* that results from the foreclosure of the Real is sought in the Imaginary and Symbolic orders. So unlike Freud's, the Lacanian 'Real' need not be outside the subject, in some sort of concrete form. For example, a Lacanian might describe a profound trauma that a subject can never hope to put into words as an effect of the Real. In the same way that the repressed memory of a trauma can lead to neurotic symptoms which threaten to dominate the subject's everyday life, so the Real is a kind of void around which both the Symbolic and the Imaginary revolve. To use Kantian terminology, the Real is the paradoxical conflation of both the condition of possibility *and* of impossibility of a given system: this is why the Real has to be, but cannot be, included.

In many ways, it is impossible to summarise Lacan himself, or Lacanian theory. His ideas ranged far and wide, and also changed a great deal during his lifetime. His form of analysis is still widely practised, particularly in France and Spain. However, his clinical approach remains controversial within more 'mainstream' forms of psychoanalysis. For example, the strategy of the 'short session', which leads to analysis stopping, often abruptly, and at any time, is incompatible with the more standard fifty-minute session. Lacanians use this method to force analysands to reflect on the meaning of their own discourse at the moment the session ends. For more orthodox Freudians, however, this practice seems to contradict the right of the 'paying customer' to expect a full 'service' measured in time. For this and other much more theoretical reasons, Lacanian analysis remains somewhat marginalised from the major institutions of psychoanalysis. Nonetheless, whatever the on-going fate of Lacanian analysis, the complexity of the theoretical vocabulary Lacan constructed, and the breadth of phenomena to which he managed to apply it (from religious paintings to courtly love, from Hegel to James Joyce), continues to provide a rich resource for the human and social sciences in general and for the analysis of consumer culture and behaviour in particular.

9 The Feminist Challenge

We have now looked at many of the important tenets of psychoanalytic theory. We have explored Sigmund Freud's seminal ideas, and we have seen how some of his successors took these ideas in new and original directions. It is now time, in the final two chapters, to acknowledge more fully the unceasingly *controversial* nature of psychoanalysis. After all, this has never been a movement that has been greeted with universal approval! From Freud's earliest publications with Breuer, the ideas of psychoanalysis have proved capable of igniting the most ferocious indignation. I have tried to highlight a few of these objections in the preceding pages. I have also pointed out that, in the concept of 'resistance', psychoanalysis often transforms the objections made against it into proofs of its own hypotheses. That is to say, the more apoplectic we get in response to the analyst's claim that we wish to murder our fathers, the more the analyst calmly replies, 'My point exactly'! Nonetheless, psychoanalysis has not been able to incorporate all of its critics in this crude way. Indeed, to be fair to psychoanalysis, it has been characterised by a mature self-critical attitude that has helped it to grow and develop into the rich diversity it displays today. However, some criticisms, by virtue of their sheer persistence, do seem to indicate some contradictions at the heart of orthodox psychoanalysis which any balanced account of the movement as a whole must address.

One such enduring criticism comes from feminists. Their objections tend to boil down to the idea that psychoanalysis is shot through with prejudices against women and against female sexuality, and that this prejudice both reflects and perpetuates the injustices of a society dominated by men. For many feminists, Freud is one of the worst culprits in a long history of the oppression of women. For other feminists, however, as we shall see, he is a pioneering thinker whose ideas can be useful in trying to conceive of a specifically feminine sexuality and identity.

What is Feminism?

Feminism is a complex international political, social and cultural movement that has a long and rich history. One might attempt to trace this history from the Amazons of ancient Greece, through Joan of Arc, and onto Mary Wollstonecraft of the eighteenth century and Simone de Beauvoir of the twentieth. And yet, such an exercise would be utterly arbitrary, as it is really impossible to circumscribe feminism's boundaries: for as long as women have been oppressed by men, there have always been individuals who have spoken out about and even fought against this oppression. The question of *how* women should fight back against male oppression has been just as complex. Should women demand equality, competing on a par with men even in predominantly male arenas? Perhaps, but doesn't this mean that the measure of success here is still 'male', and thus that men have already 'won' by pre-determining the very terms of the battle of the sexes? So is it better to pursue specifically female *alternatives* to these masculine norms, alternatives built upon the special traits of femininity? Perhaps, but isn't there a danger in this approach of essentialising women, that is, of reducing them to stereotypical traits like intuition, emotional sensitivity, and maternal instinct, etc.?

Even if we try to impose a more restrictive *political* definition of feminism, we are still confronted by great diversity. For example, some feminists are fairly militant Marxists who follow Marx and Engels in believing that the family is the first form of slavery, and that the first mode of subjugation in all societies is that of women by men. For these Marxist feminists, the problem of male domination is absolutely tied up with capitalism, so that the solution to the problems about which feminists complain has to be revolution, and the transition to Communism. However, there are also feminists at the other end of the political spectrum who feel that the real problem faced by women is poverty and lack of opportunity. Such feminists may argue that the only way to improve the lot of women around the world is to *spread* capitalism, not overthrow it, so that women can enjoy the same employment opportunities and income potential as men. Still other feminists would argue that what women actually suffer from is the lack of a voice in the male-dominated arenas of representational politics. Clearly, these feminists believe that a greater number of representatives in, for example, the British Houses of Parliament, would enable a greater push for top-down change through governmental policies and institutional reform. These three types of feminists might in fact share hardly any common ground at all, yet they are still feminists!

One simple way to make sense of the complexity of feminism is to divide it into first, second and third-wave feminisms. This has the advantage of sketching, albeit very roughly, the recent history of feminism. First-wave feminism refers to the early days of an organised and politicised feminist movement formed in England in the mid to late eighteenth century, a time when the gap between men and women in terms of rights and privileges was enormous. Remarkable women like Mary Wollstonecraft and Bessie Rayner Parkes described the plight of women and applied pressure to improve access to education and professional jobs, and to strengthen custody rights as well as property rights within marriage. There was also a concerted campaign to secure the vote for women, but this was a long time coming in many European countries and in the United States.

Second-wave feminism refers to the explosion of feminist activism that coincided with the sexual revolution and black civil rights movements in the 1960s. It was characterised by direct action as well as intellectual and cultural production which challenged prevailing stereotypes about women. A famous slogan which typifies much of second-wave feminism is 'the personal is the political', which conveys the widespread attempt both to change the domestic and social situations of women, and to imagine an alternative way of doing politics which might improve women's situations. However, second-wave feminism was also always characterised by great diversity, encompassing black, lesbian, liberal and radical feminisms, so that even at its most dynamic, feminism was hardly a coherent programme.

The third-wave feminism that emerged in the 1980s represents an attempt to react to the apparent gains that some women – at least in developed countries – have gained in the last half century, which range from improved political representation to the greater potential for high-powered careers. The dilemmas for contemporary feminists are, after all, rather different than for their Suffragette precursors! Where first-wave feminists could neither vote nor enter certain professions (such as medicine), third-wave feminists struggle to balance careers with raising children. This may be a nice problem to have, in that it is born of a certain privilege that was not there previously, but it is still a problem (one that has its legal dimension in things like maternity leave and return to work policies).

Needless to say, such divisions are inordinately clumsy, and one must always bear in mind that the goals of second-wave feminism have not all been fulfilled, so that many battles continue to be fought. For example, despite all the privileges of being born into a well developed Western country, a baby girl is proportionally still more likely to earn less when she grows up than her male counter-part. Moreover, in many less developed countries, Third World women are doubly exploited, firstly by the demands of a fairly primitive capitalism which can lead them into conditions of sweatshop labour, and secondly, by their cultures, whose traditions can often be fiercely and stubbornly prejudicial to women. From whichever angle you look at it, women still do not enjoy complete equality with men.

These descriptions should emphasise that what feminism has been or could be is less important (and less urgent) than that it continues in its various guises today. Despite its diversity, however, let us be reductionist for a moment, and claim that just about all forms of feminism include two basic elements: criticism of male-dominated societies and advocacy of equality (of access, of rights, of privileges, etc.) for women. As part of the first, most feminisms share the claim that almost all societies, but particularly modern societies, are what is termed 'patriarchal'. The word comes from Greek, with *patria* meaning 'father' (*pater* in Latin) and *archê* meaning 'rule' or 'command'. As the word *patria* indicates, the concept of patriarchy really has as its underlying conceptual metaphor the family, with the father definitely at the 'head of the family': it is the 'law of the father' that rules the house, and, by extension, society. Indeed, many anthropologists have used the term 'patriarchy' to describe so-called primitive societies, whose structures, rituals and practices are nearly always organised around men. However, the way that feminists use the notion of 'patriarchy' is a little more broad, in that it refers to the disproportionate attribution of social power to men, over and above, and at the expense of, women. Feminists who object to patriarchy object to the unequal division of power along gender lines, with men always getting the lion's share of influence, privilege and prestige, while women are little more than second-class citizens (if, in fact, they qualify as citizens at all).

Perhaps all this talk of families, fathers, and the law of the father already suggests why individual feminists in particular, and the feminist movement in general, have long engaged in a productive dialogue with psychoanalysis. However, psychoanalysis proves to be as divisive in the field of feminist politics and theory as it has been in those of psychology and social theory.

Feminism and Psychoanalysis

In addressing the collaborations and confrontations between feminism and psychoanalysis, perhaps it is best to begin by invoking the idea of a love-hate relationship. This is because two apparently incompatible approaches to psychoanalysis divide today's feminisms more or less in two. On the one hand, there are those who 'hate' psychoanalysis because they think of it as little more than *a normative endorsement of patriarchy*. Secondly, however, there are those feminists who 'love' psychoanalysis, as it were, because they can see in it a useful *descriptive analysis of patriarchy*. So there are those feminists who think that psychoanalysis is very much part of the problem (that it is instrumental in the oppression of women), and there are those that think it merely describes the problem with incomparable clarity, and is therefore of profound value. Let's look at these two approaches.

If feminists concentrate on the first, 'normative' approach to psychoanalysis, they deploy what might be called an 'external critique'. That is to say, they very deliberately position themselves *outside* the ideas and claims of psychoanalysis, of which they are profoundly sceptical, in order to show how it constructs arguments that lead directly to the oppression of women through both the practice of therapy, and through the wider dissemination of prejudicial ideas in society as a whole. Such an external critique tends to follow roughly the following argumentative structure:

1. Freud was himself a sexist patriarch: this *ad hominem* approach employs biographical as well as theoretical textual evidence to demonstrate that as an individual, Freud was typical of his time, his

gender, and his social class, in the assumptions he made about women.

2. Freudianism defines femininity from a biased (male) point of view: this pursues the supposed impact of Freud's own prejudices on his theoretical work, concentrating, for example, on the male-centred narrative of sexual and social development in Freud's account of the Oedipus Complex.
3. Psychoanalysis is a *tool* of patriarchy: it follows from the bias within Freudianism, and from its implementation in the therapeutic setting, that psychoanalysis as a whole actually imposes the prejudices it redescribes as scientific facts. This means, in essence, that the female analysand will be *more* oppressed after analysis than she was before it.
4. Psychoanalysis perpetuates a narrow view of femininity: because Freudianism only explains female sexuality as a negative relationship with male sexuality, it is argued that it constrains femininity to two roles – either a marital role as a wife, or a maternal role as a mother. Neither role allows women to be women on their own terms.

Evidently, these are very serious accusations. Indeed, as we shall see in a moment, elements of these criticisms crop up again in the 'internal critiques' of those feminists who are actually sympathetic to psychoanalysis. However, these four argumentative steps of the 'external' type are characterised by a founding *rejection* of the basic tenets of psychoanalysis, such as the notion of the unconscious and the importance of repression in social life. According to this 'normative' understanding, the 'unconscious' would merely be one theoretical fiction within the patriarchal mythology of psychoanalysis, deployed as an instrument of male domination.

As we have noted before, psychoanalysis does have its normative dimension, insofar as its therapeutic goal is to 'normalise' people, often into more socially acceptable gender roles. That is to say, an hysterical woman who comes to analysis may be said to be avoiding her own sexual impulses, and a successful therapeutic outcome would be her reintegration, *as* a woman, into the very society that imposes unfair, because male-centred, standards of repression on her feminine sexuality. The psychoanalyst becomes, on this account, a kind of behavioural policeman, who brings the errant woman back into line with the patriarchal norm of femininity.

In contrast, those feminists who perform an 'internal critique' fundamentally accept the basic tenets of psychoanalysis – such as the existence of the unconscious, repression, and the dynamic importance of the libido – but take specific issue with the way these tenets have been used to describe female sexuality and identity. Their critique is 'internal' to psychoanalysis to the extent that it accepts most of the discipline's postulates (as we shall see, many feminists of this kind are themselves practising psychoanalysts). Such feminists are likely to accept aspects of points 1, 2 and 4 above, but they are less likely to endorse in any simple way point 3, which is that psychoanalysis is *necessarily* patriarchal. Indeed, rather than seeing psychoanalysis as a normative endorsement of patriarchy, they see it as the best theoretical description available of the actual *workings* of patriarchy. Just as it is a basic principle of battle that you should 'know your enemy', these feminists argue that psychoanalysis can help oppressed women to know *how* they are oppressed and, therefore, it can describe ways of combating oppression. Admittedly, this line between normative and descriptive aspects of psychoanalytic theory and practice is somewhat blurry, particularly in the area of clinical practice. Nevertheless, these feminists are motivated by a more optimistic hope for psychoanalysis, including the idea that it can contribute to the political project of the women's liberation movement (as more than a mere straw man to be ritually knocked down).

The rationale is that psychoanalysis can be helpful to feminism in two different but complementary ways: as an existing vocabulary for feminist critiques of patriarchy; and as a vocabulary which can be changed from the inside to provide an improved and perhaps an emancipatory description of femininity. Psychoanalysis is therefore not to be dismissed or discounted, but used as a valuable tool in the fight against patriarchy.

How can Psychoanalysis be useful to Feminism?

As just one indication of how psychoanalysis can be useful to feminism, we can consider an important distinction made by both 'external' and 'internal' feminists, a distinction between 'sex' and 'gender'. In everyday language, these words are used in a fairly lazy way, so that they seem pretty much interchangeable. For example, whilst filling out a form for a job or a visa, we might be asked to indicate either our sex or our gender, often with an 'M' or an 'F'. Yet for feminists, these are really quite different things.

Sex is a thoroughly biological category. It relates primarily to the reproductive organs that indicate whether an individual is a male or a female of the species. In this sense, it is generally very clear cut, because it is demonstrable and observable. In contrast, many feminists claim that gender is a cultural construction. That is, it is something that the values and norms of a society impose on us, often so effectively that we mistake it for something thoroughly 'natural'. To take a crude example, masculine genders are already being imposed on children when expectant mothers, who discover that their unborn child is male, paint the walls of the nursery blue, and buy bibs with pictures of cars and footballers on them, and, a few years later, guns and soldiers for them to play with. Girls, of course, often get pink bedrooms and bibs with flowers on and dolls to play with! Although this example is rather caricatured, it does demonstrate that the world into which we arrive as infants is already distinguished by a clear gender divide. As we grow up, we adorn ourselves with 'signifiers' (to use Saussure's term) of our genders: our clothes, our taste in music, our leisure activities, the way we relate to our friends. Unlike sex, which is more obviously bodily and therefore relatively fixed (notwithstanding surgical interventions), gender is fluid and unfixed.

Indeed, one famous gender theorist, Judith Butler, takes this argument to the extreme by collapsing the very distinction between sex and gender, effectively making everything gender.[1] She argues that all gender and sexual identity is thoroughly *performed*: we wear it, we speak it, we gesture it, we act it out in our sexual and emotional lives as actors perform lines on the stage. This means that there is in fact nothing 'natural' or inevitable about it, that it is *only* a social construction. For some feminists, this argument doesn't take into account what it is like to, as it were, live in a woman's body, which does indeed have its own specificity and which perhaps shapes, in turn, processes of social construction (that is, a body may be subjected to social 'discipline', but the contours of the body still govern the kind of 'discipline' to which it can be subjected). Arguably, Butler, as a lesbian Queer Theorist, has a particular agenda in this argument, which is to demonstrate that heterosexuality is itself the result of a repressed homosexual urge. Indeed, this is precisely where psychoanalysis comes to her aid, as many psychoanalysts advocate Freud's founding insight into the 'constitutive bisexuality' of the human being.

So although this debate about the role of the body within feminist theory remains fierce, what is important for us is that it has been enabled largely by Freud, and by Freud's intervention into the theorisation of sexuality. As you will recall from chapter 4, Freud's analysis of homosexuality, or 'inversion' as he called it, immediately indicated the radical mobility of desire. We have a libidinal instinct, he argued, but the objects toward which that libido is directed can change (witness the 'contingent invert'). Moreover, the very aims toward which it tends can be extremely varied, as evidenced by the polymorphous perversity of infants, and by the fetishism of perverts. Although Freud did not make the distinction between sex and gender himself, his broadly biological outlook nonetheless pushed him towards an insight into the contingency of 'object-choice', or what we might normally call 'sexual persuasion'. Furthermore, his discussion of the 'camp' and 'butch' behavioural traits of certain partners in same-sex relationships demonstrated an intuition about the performative dimension

[1] Butler, Judith. *Gender Trouble: Feminism and the Subversion of Identity* (London: Routledge, 1999).

of what subsequent feminists would indeed call gender. And, of course, Freud's general emphasis on the emergence of subjectivity from social repression already prefigures the more political side of Judith Butler's argument, which is that, if gender is performed, and women are oppressed, then the impoverished nature of gender roles enforced on women by social repression is a major part of their plight *as* women.

Because psychoanalysis has always paid such close attention to the play between bodily needs, sexuality, and the repressive force of social mores, it is peculiarly well-placed to contribute to these important debates.

Julia Kristeva: a Psychoanalytic Feminist

Let us now look at an example of such an 'internal' critique of orthodox psychoanalysis, by briefly considering some of the ideas put forward by the philosopher and psychoanalyst, Julia Kristeva.

Although born in Bulgaria, Kristeva is now a French citizen who writes in French (note the present tense: we have now moved forward enough in time to be speaking of *living* psychoanalytic theorists). She is herself a practising analyst. Her re-workings of psychoanalytic theory are powerfully shaped by her diverse interests, which include Kleinianism, linguistics, literature (particularly the *nouveau roman*), and philosophy. In actual fact, Kristeva is rather reluctant to call herself a feminist, and she occasionally has less than flattering things to say about aspects of the feminist movement. Nonetheless, by concentrating on just three aspects of her rich body of work, it is possible to pin, albeit in a qualified manner, the label of 'feminist' on her intellectual inclinations, if not her espoused political commitments. These three aspects are the *chora*, the semiotic, and 'herethics'.

Kristeva takes the concept of the 'chora' from a work by the Greek philosopher, Plato, called the *Timaeus*. Plato's age-old problem in the *Timaeus*, which physicists are still grappling with today, is how the universe began, or how something emerged out of nothing. In the *Timaeus*, Plato constructs a mythological cosmology of the origin of everything, and it is in this context that he uses the word 'chora'. On a literal level, it means something like 'receptacle', yet Plato describes it with reference to the 'womb', to 'wetnurses', and to 'containers' as well as 'producers'. Evidently, he is struggling here to describe a passage from non-existence to existence, with the *chora* acting as the space that somehow precedes and yet paves the way for life. What has this got to do with psychoanalysis, you may well ask? Kristeva transposes Plato's peculiar usage of *chora* to the psychoanalytic equivalent of the moment before the universe began. She transposes it to the pre-Oedipal child, who is not yet a differentiated entity (as we saw with Klein) and cannot yet use language, and who is therefore on the brink of the universe of subjectivity.

Because Kristeva is influenced by Klein, she thinks of this pre-Oedipal period as having important connections to the mother. Yet this is not the mother in any simple sense, because the *chora* pre-exists language and, therefore, the label 'mother' cannot be applied yet. Rather, just as Klein emphasised the originary relationship to the part-object of the breast, which continues to affect us in later life, so Kristeva emphasises this period of the *chora* and the impact it has on, specifically, communication. Kristeva argues that although the baby cannot speak, this does not mean it cannot communicate. As baby-sitters know only too well, babies can cry and scream, as well as gurgle and coo. In this non-symbolic way, babies can communicate their emotional status (whether they are hungry or happy). For Kristeva – who, like Lacan, is extremely interested in linguistics and the literarinesss of language – the *chora* represents a pre-Oedipal (pre-Symbolic in Lacan's vocabulary) arrangement of the drives that impacts on communication. Thus, just as the Platonic *chora* paves the way for the beginnings of life, so the Kristevan *chora* paves the way for the acquisition of symbolic language and the birth of subjectivity. The fact that Kristeva lays such stress on the mother and on the feminine nature of the *chora* is surely not insignificant for feminism.

This immediately brings us to Kristeva's idea of the 'semiotic', which she contrasts with the symbolic. The symbolic basically refers to language as we normally conceive of it, which is to say, as a formal means of expression reliant upon laws of syntax, grammar and propositional logic which pertain to states of affairs in the world, usually amenable to some kind of proof. In contrast, the 'semiotic', in Kristeva's rather idiosyncratic use of this word (which should not be conflated too quickly with the science of semiotics), refers to *non-linguistic aspects of language that express drives and affects*. Thus, the semiotic level contains rhythms and sounds that can convey powerful yet indefinable emotions (recall the intense emotion that the baby conveys in its supposedly 'meaningless' cry). Perhaps a simple way to visualise this contrast between the symbolic and the semiotic is to picture a scale sliding between two poles:

(Symbolic) **(Semiotic)**
Mathematics◄——— Prose◄———————►Poetry ———————►Music

Here, we can see that at the extreme end of the symbolic pole is mathematical language, because that is the most 'self-identical' language conceivable, with 1 always standing for 1 (so that 1 plus 1 always equals 2). At the most semiotic extreme, on the other hand, is music, because music can affect us very profoundly on an emotional level, yet it cannot really be said to represent anything. For example, classical music can induce deep melancholy, or fill us with unbounded joy, yet it doesn't do this by telling a tragic or uplifting story. Part way between the two halves, and echoing Kristeva's interest in literature, prose is placed on the side of the symbolic because it is proportionally more 'representational' (it has characters, scenes, historical backdrops, and so on) than poetry, which deserves to be considered as more semiotic, because it utilises precisely the musical aspects of language that rhetorical theory designates as metre, assonance, alliteration and so on.

However, we must issue a *caveat emptor* (or buyer beware) here, because Kristeva's point, above and beyond these binary oppositions, is that *all* communication must have both symbolic and semiotic components. The symbolic and semiotic are like the *recto* and *verso* of the same sheet of paper. The radical consequence, which the neatness of our scale elides, is that even so-called normal communication has an indelible semiotic element, and that this can give expression to the semiotic chora, as that aspect of language in which bodily drives and desires can find affective expression.

From a feminist perspective this is very significant, because the symbolic and semiotic aspects of language are, according to Kristeva, masculine and feminine respectively. Just as Lacan adapts Freud's Oedipus Complex by arguing that entry into the Symbolic is the moment when a certain *jouissance* has to be relinquished in order to subject oneself to the 'Law of the Father', so Kristeva argues that the symbolic specifically represses the feminine semiotic. That is, the symbolic denies expression to the *jouissance* attached to the maternal body but, as the semiotic *chora,* it irrupts nonetheless in the form of cadence, physical gesture, vocal rhythm and so on. This is why, in her own clinical practice, Kristeva sometimes makes use of song with her patients: she believes that the semiotic qualities of music, breath, voice and rhythm etc. can allow expression of affects normally inexpressible in the symbolic mode of language. For women particularly, this may allow them to 'get in touch' with a certain inner femininity normally denied them. This is also why Kristeva is so interested in the avant-garde poetry of writers like Céline and Stéphane Mallarmé (note that these happen to be men, which just shows that biological sex is not the issue here), and in the literary theories of thinkers like Mikhail Bakhtin and Roland Barthes. Poetry, like song, can give voice to the semiotic *chora.*

Indeed, it was this belief in the expressive possibilities of poetic language for women in particular that led to the wider movement called *écriture féminine* in France. This experimental form of expression was intended to break out of the restrictive masculine symbolic mode in order to access a positive femininity. One could read this movement from Judith Butler's perspective, of gender-as-social-construction. On this account, *écriture féminine* would be an intervention into the contingent gender roles made available to women by society, giving them a position alternative to the dominant male stereotype of femininity. However, this is not how Kristeva sees things, for the whole point of her psychoanalytic theory is that the embodied nature of existence cannot be sidestepped. The semiotic represents the drives and affects of the (female) body, and the imbrication of desire into language.

The importance of the female body in Kristeva's thought becomes even more obvious in her idea of 'herethics'. As the term itself indicates, this is her attempt to describe a specifically feminine ethics. Echoing the second-wave feminist dictum that 'the personal is the political', Kristeva builds her argument out of her own experience of pregnancy. Her fundamental claim is that the relationship between mother and child prior to birth can provide a kind of model for a feminist ethics. In addressing the philosophical issue of ethics, Kristeva is not actually straying all that far from psychoanalysis. After all, the two disciplines have in common a deep interest in intersubjectivity, which is to say, in how people relate to one another. From the point of view of psychoanalysis, a genetic account of the emergence of subjectivity in an always already social and socialising context necessarily involves an account of human interrelations. What else is Freud's description of the transition from primary to secondary narcissism, with a necessary passage through identification? How else can we describe Klein's emphasis on introjection and projection? Isn't this exactly what Lacan was getting at when he theorised the role of the Other in the order of the Symbolic? In a similar fashion then, ethics concerns itself with how the self relates to others. In particular, ethics asks how a self is able to relate to the Other as a fellow sentient human being with feelings and needs etc.. The Christian principle that we should 'do unto others as we would have them do unto us' is an ethical principle because it encourages the recognition of the equal and intrinsic value of the experiences and feelings of others. By contrast, what psychoanalysis might describe as the pathological condition of psychopathy, and what a certain theologically inflected ethics might describe as Evil, involves treating other subjects as mere objects.

So this question of the relation between self and other is common to both psychoanalysis and ethics, yet Kristeva uses the fact of pregnancy to blur this very distinction. In beautifully poetic language, she describes intense waves of emotion washing over her during pregnancy, which were not randomly hormonal, but powerfully invested in the child developing in her womb. In other words, Kristeva experienced profound love for her unborn child. Yet the boundary between self and other, which is normally a condition of all forms of love (other than primary narcissism), is of course thoroughly absent in this instance, because the baby is, as it were, an Other within. Kristeva has never 'met' this nascent person, yet feels an overwhelming and utterly unconditional love for them. It is a love that bypasses the prescriptive form of morality ('thou shalt not …') which is based on a sense of duty, as well as that reward-based form of morality that coerces ethical behaviour through a combination of threats (eternal damnation) and promises (eternal bliss) to be realised sometime in the future.

For Kristeva, it is also significant that this blurring between self and other during pregnancy has nothing to do with the symbolic dimension of language. The bond experienced during pregnancy is indescribable because it predates language and the symbolic, occupying instead an embodied semiotic relationship with the mother's body. It is this that begins to explain the punning term with which Kristeva chooses to describe this mother-child relation – 'herethics'. This neologism works rather better in the French. It combines *hérétique* (heretical) with *éthique* (ethics), and thus conveys the two sides of what Kristeva is proposing. The mother-child ethical model is heretical because it breaks the paternal 'Law of the Father' which, as Lacan claimed, organises the Symbolic (the religious resonance of the word heretical also refers back to Freud's connection between the internalised father of the super-ego and the image of an admonishing God). It is ethical because it concerns the traditional ethical problem of the relation between self and other, albeit by apparently collapsing that relation into a very specific, physiological phenomenon.

In fact, many feminists in the Anglophone world have reacted to these notions with shouts of 'essentialism!' (something of a four-letter word amongst feminists). One can understand their reasoning. After all, isn't Kristeva simply repeating what Freud had already said, which is that women are really and truly women only when they are mothers, and when they are using their bodies to make babies? Perhaps we shouldn't assume that ethical theories must make universal claims, yet it is still pertinent to point out that the experience of pregnancy is hardly open to all. This is true not only from a male perspective (unlike Arnold Schwarzenegger in the film *Junior*, men are currently unlikely to experience pregnancy), but also from the perspective of women who can't have children, as well as women who simply do not want children. For many feminists, the stereotype of the fertile mother (Earth) is one they are trying to escape. However, the objections to Kristeva's ideas are divided along predictable lines, with the Anglophone world on one side, and continental Europe on the other.

As we have already seen, feminists in the Anglophone world tend to emphasise the idea of gender as social construction, and they therefore concern themselves very closely with practical issues which empirically constrain the expression and freedom of women. For example, feminists in America currently campaign around the extremely contentious issue of abortion. Continental European feminists, particularly those influenced by French thought, are much more philosophically inclined, so that people like Kristeva and the Belgian-born philosopher, Luce Irigaray, point their feminist fingers at the 'phallocentric' history of Western metaphysics. However, like most such divisions, this supposed divide is more false than true. Firstly, continental feminists are by no means disengaged from activism on practical issues. Secondly, it is a prejudice of the Anglo-saxon tradition to view this concern with philosophy as high-minded, bookish, and irrelevant to the 'front-line'. After all, philosophy has been one of the most important places where images of woman have been 'forged': the conceptual heritage from philosophy powerfully shapes even the 'pragmatic' formulation of policies which directly impact on the lives of women today. These are therefore cultural, rather than conceptual, contrasts, and in fact progressive feminism on both sides of the Atlantic demonstrates a creative deployment of both approaches.

10 For and Against Psychoanalysis

Let us close this introduction to the major tenets and thinkers of psychoanalytic theory by assessing some arguments for and against the movement as a whole. This is important because the controversial nature of psychoanalysis has produced almost as many pages of vicious opprobrium as of passionate advocacy: discounting either body of writing would be unacceptably partial.

It is also important to reflect the somewhat reduced fortunes of psychoanalytic therapy today. Concentrating on the *ideas* of psychoanalysis should not disguise the fact that, as a branch of psychology, its peak undoubtedly came in the troubled post-war years of the late 1940s and 1950s. Today, it forms a significant yet hardly central backdrop to psychodynamic approaches within mainstream psychology (which are in their turn largely overshadowed by behavioural approaches). Indeed, within the Anglophone academic world in particular, Freud is more likely to appear on a course about the *history* of psychology, than on a practical course about contemporary therapeutic techniques. Even though clinical psychoanalysis continues to be very popular in certain cosmopolitan locations such as Paris, New York and Buenos Aires, from the perspective of Freud's own *medical* ambitions, these are disappointing exceptions to the rule: it is therefore still possible to argue that the psychoanalytic star has waned since the latter half of the twentieth century.

On the other hand, and despite his best efforts, psychoanalysis was always bigger than Freud himself. Consequently, if the star of (scientifically respectable) therapeutic psychoanalysis has perhaps dimmed, psychoanalysis as an important tool within a venerable tradition of critique within the humanities – which would include figures such as Kant, Hegel and Marx – arguably burns brighter than ever today. One might even go further by arguing that the relative marginalisation of psychoanalytic theory is actually symptomatic of the *increasing* importance of a critical psychoanalytic social theory in today's consumer culture. The movement of psychoanalysis out of departments of psychology and into departments of literature, cultural studies and even continental philosophy describes a movement away from the harder sciences and towards the softer social sciences. Even if this contradicts Freud's original hope for his discipline, it nonetheless represents the dominant intellectual role played by the movement in the twenty-first century. This fairly strong claim for psychoanalytic theory makes an analysis of the arguments for and against the movement even more imperative.

Arguments For Psychoanalysis

The modes of critique to which psychoanalysis has been subjected, from its inception to the present day, can, despite their variety, be schematically divided into four categories: personal, theoretical, political, and ethical.

Personal

The personal approach indulges attacks on Freud primarily as the founding father of psychoanalysis. We addressed this tendency in the preceding chapter, in which we encountered the 'external' critiques of feminists who claim that Freud was himself a sexist patriarch. Throughout, we have explained (but not excused) these predispositions as a product of Freud's cultural milieu, class standing and historical context. It is to place too much faith in the universal nature of rationality to expect Freud to think in absolute disjuncture from the assumptions of his time. A potentially more devastating *ad hominem* argument, however, comes from Richard Webster, in his provocatively titled but meticulously researched *Why Freud Was Wrong*.[1] Deploying the personal approach to good effect, Webster argues that Freud's intense ambition eclipsed his scientific objectivity. In other words, Freud was so much the blinkered careerist that he discarded the measured caution befitting a genuine scientist.

This argument finds support in three key incidents from the earliest days of psychoanalysis. Firstly, there was the so-called 'cocaine episode' of 1884. During this period, when the precise effects of this new drug were still unknown, Freud had experimented with taking it himself. He then prescribed it for his patients, and was so impressed by the results, both in himself and in the well-being of those in his care, that he published an article entitled 'On Cocaine' in a respected Viennese journal. The article ascribed miraculous anaesthetic properties to the drug and, indeed, came close to describing it as a panacea for all ills. Whilst evidence of the addictive and harmful effects of cocaine were not initially available to Freud, such evidence emerged rapidly in the wake of his article. At first – and this is Webster's point about ambition getting in the way of reason – Freud scoffed at the criticisms of his putative wonder drug, whose curative properties he continued, for quite a time, to laud. Later, Freud's personal biographer, Ernest Jones, would put this obstinacy down to the effects of the drug on Freud himself. This must remain mere speculation, yet Freud was eventually forced to concede that cocaine wasn't the unqualified good he had described, and that he had made a professional mistake.

Secondly, and much more seriously for the now canonical mythology of psychoanalysis, it seems likely that Freud (and Josef Breuer) may have

[1] Webster, Richard. *Why Freud Was Wrong: Sin, Science and Psychoanalysis* (London: HarperCollins, 1996).

exaggerated the effectiveness of the 'talking cure' in the seminal case of 'Anna O'. This was a pseudonym for a female patient who suffered from severe hysterical symptoms, including periodic paralysis, loss of the power of speech, and a persistent nervous cough. In their *Studies on Hysteria* of 1895, Freud and Breuer claimed to have completely cured this baffling range of ailments through their novel 'cathartic method'. For many disciples of psychoanalysis today, Anna O. was both the first psychoanalytic patient in history and the first irrefutable illustration of its therapeutic powers. However, years after the account of her case in *Studies on Hysteria*, Ernest Jones took the unusual step of revealing, in his biography of Freud, the real name of the troubled young woman: she was one Bertha Pappenheim. This information enabled the archivally assiduous to track down the fate of the real individual, so long hidden behind the pseudonym. Subsequent medical records proved that Bertha Pappenheim went on to spend time in a sanatorium *after* her psychoanalytic treatment with Freud and Breuer. Indeed, she continued to suffer from some symptoms for the rest of her life (although others never reappeared). The cathartic cure, it seems, was not as complete as Freud and Breuer had claimed.

Thirdly, Freud himself came to view one of his own early theoretical positions with sharp regret. This related to his so-called 'seduction theory', which pre-dated the fully elaborated theory of psychosexual development as expounded in his *Three Essays on the Theory of Sexuality*. At this time, Freud was focussing much of his attention on the phenomenon of repression, yet his paradigmatic model remained that of traumatic amnesia. Thus, his aetiology of hysteria, which he quickly determined to have sexual origins, initially included the assumption that symptoms stemmed from repressed memories of *actual* sexual abuse. As one can readily imagine, such supposed revelations caused intense anguish both for the individuals who came to Freud for help, and for their families, some of whose members were suddenly accused of being child molesters. While Freud's later 'discovery' of unconscious fantasies led him to view the 'seduction theory' as mistaken, one could argue that his new stance was not much of an improvement. After all, did he not go too far in the other direction, potentially dismissing genuine recollections of sexual abuse that emerged during therapeutic regression as mere Oedipal fantasy? At both extremes, one could claim that it was Freud's own zeal to 'prove' his theories that steamrollered over individual needs.

Theoretical

These personal attacks on Freud merge with more theoretically orientated assaults on Freudianism, many of which concentrate on their common claim to scientific respectability. Thus, it is an easy but also perfectly logical step to claim that Freud's burning ambition got in the way of his scientific objectivity. For one thing, he broke a cardinal rule of a certain view of science, by taking himself as his own object of study. Even though Freud would come to advocate a detached and professional relationship between analyst and analysand, in his earliest speculations about the nature of the unconscious he was nonetheless his own experimental guinea-pig. He subjected himself to sustained self-analysis by exploring his darkest recesses for what he regarded as reliable psychological data, and it was on this inner journey that he discovered the infamous Oedipus Complex. He then extrapolated from these data a universal psychic drama, assuming, of course, that all our minds would be similar to his! This *modus operandi* is clearly very different from the image of the scientist examining his object of study through a microscope, and from an appropriate distance.

There is also the issue of the rather unscientific influences (by today's standards) upon which Freud drew in formulating psychoanalytic doctrine. In fact, Webster combines the personal and theoretical modes of criticism by arguing that, as a personality, Freud was prone to extreme hero-worship: particularly as a young man, he would attach himself to pioneering intellectuals whose fallibility he then refused to admit. This in itself impeded his judgement, but the problem was compounded by the heroes whom Freud chose to worship, whose theories do not stand up to scrutiny today. Two figures in particular must be mentioned in this regard: Jean Martin Charcot and Wilhelm Fliess.

Jean Martin Charcot is generally considered the founder of modern neurology. Freud studied with him at the *Salpêtrièr* Hospital in Paris at a time when Charcot's reputation across Europe was immense. However, according to Webster, Charcot's most important discoveries were already behind him when Freud came to work with him. Worse, Charcot was beginning to be led astray, scientifically, by his interest in a strange phenomenon – hypnotism. Charcot had already gathered a number of 'hysterics' in the *Salpêtrièr* Hospital and he soon began experimenting on these unfortunates with hypnosis, even organising public demonstrations of its strange effects upon them. Using hypnotic techniques, Charcot could induce dramatic seizures at will, or suspend previously incessant tremors and tics. The Paris public flocked to this bizarre spectacle, and Freud was just as impressed as everyone else. Hypnotism is significant in the pre-history of psychoanalysis because it suggested to Freud the importance of psychological factors in physical symptoms. However, Webster makes the crucial point that, interpreted with modern medical knowledge, Charcot's own case notes about the 'hysterics' housed at the *Salpêtrièr* Hospital strongly indicate that most of them would today be diagnosed as either epileptics, or victims of traumatic brain injury. That is to say, their problems related to physical lesions on the brain, rather than to faulty psychological mechanisms. Webster claims that Charcot's mistake (confusing the physiological with the psychological) became Freud's mistake, and that Freud magnified it enormously in his postulation of the unconscious.

If Charcot was a deservedly famous physician who, in his later career, took a wrong turning, Wilhelm Fliess made nothing *but* wrong turnings from today's scientific point of view. Freud came under Fliess's sway after his time with Charcot (they exchanged many letters between 1897 and 1902), during a period, in fact, when the very pillars of psychoanalysis were being established. Yet even in his own time, Fliess's ideas were decidedly oddball. He was fascinated by the connections between evolutionary biology and individual development. Post-Darwin, this was not unusual, and it certainly influenced Freud (for example, in his theory of psychosexual development, where his distinction between 'phylogenesis' and 'ontogenesis' was taken *tout court* from Fliess). However, while Fliess's avowed aim was to make biology as mathematical as physics, this rational aspiration was pursued in a bizarrely irrational way. Thus, he extrapolated from the average number of days in a woman's menstrual cycle to speculate about a cosmological equation that governed the rhythms of all life! He called this 'vital periodicity', and made some extremely grandiose claims about its implications. Indeed, the occult 'science' of numerology became central to Fliess's approach to evolution. As a rhino-laryngologist by training, which is to say, a nose and throat specialist, Fliess also posited a 'nasal reflex neurosis' which presupposed some kind of connection between the nose and the genitals! Perhaps most alarmingly, he claimed to be able to cure neurotic ailments connected with this 'nasal reflex' through surgical intervention into the sinuses – an operation he carried out several times, at least once with tragic results. The albeit indirect influence of these ideas on Freud, at exactly the time he was consolidating what we now know as psychoanalysis, hardly strengthens its claim to legitimacy. Webster argues that neither Charcot nor Fliess were heroes that Freud should have admired, let alone allowed to influence his own work.

These criticisms apply to the early years of a still nascent psychoanalysis. Yet much theoretical scorn has been poured upon the fundamental interpretative techniques of established clinical psychoanalysis too. The basic claim here is that the so-called 'talking cure' is a profoundly unscientific approach. Of course, this depends on which understanding of science is at work. Yet surely all science has to assume that the language it uses to describe phenomena does not interfere with those phenomena: scientific language must aspire to neutrality. The same cannot be said of psychoanalysis, which *intervenes* in its object of study. Indeed, some claim that there is an intrinsic violence in the way that classical Freudianism reduces experiences to a pre-existing theoretical edifice. Even Freud's own descriptions of his clinical procedure suggest that there may be something in this criticism. In encouraging patients to open up to free association, Freud requires that the analyst is guided in identifying 'correct' associations by the alterations induced in the patient, while all other material is to be ignored. Webster points out that if Freud's patients were suffering from physiological, not psychological, complaints, these associations would probably coincide with the normal ebb and flow of symptoms typical of most somatic ailments. When the symptoms abated for merely physical, chemical reasons, Freud assumed that it was the power of his own intervention that was having a therapeutic effect. He also assumed that whatever memories or associations the analysand was recounting at the time of this apparent improvement were the ones that pertained most closely to the specific repression causing all the trouble. In this sense, Freud attributed causality to a merely incidental factor. More fundamentally, his technique was not objective because it could seek (and, not surprisingly, find) only what it was predisposed to look for.

The philosopher Karl Popper has made a particularly cogent critique of this aspect of psychoanalysis.[2] He argues that what really separates the scientific approach from myths, religions and fanciful forms of metaphysics, is that science is very explicit about the empirical events or observations whose occurrence would invalidate a particular scientific proposition. To take an example, if the third law of thermodynamics says that all systems must lose energy, then the invention of a genuine perpetual motion machine would prove that the third law of thermodynamics is false (or at least not universally true). Popper calls this the 'criterion of falsifiability', and argues that all scientific disciplines must apply this test to themselves to be truly scientific. According to Popper, psychoanalysis fails this test because it does not explicitly describe an empirical state of affairs that would disprove its own assumptions. Indeed, he claims that psychoanalysis implicitly 'explains' everything, meaning that it isn't really making a scientific truth-claim at all. Rather, it is a very clever interpretative system that is able to re-describe almost any phenomena in its own terms. Just as the 'prophecies' of the sixteenth century astrologer, Nostradamus, *seem* to be able to predict the future because they are open-ended enough to be continually applied to the present, so notions like 'penis-envy' and 'castration anxiety' *seem* to describe all sorts of emotions and behaviours because they are, hermeneutically, extremely promiscuous. Popper does not claim that psychoanalysis is worthless, simply that it is not scientific.

Popper is really talking about the philosophy of science here, but the *practice* of contemporary science also challenges psychoanalysis. For

[2] Popper, Karl. *Conjectures and Refutations: The Growth of Scientific Knowledge* (London: Routledge, 1989).

example, neuroscience has often had an antagonistic relationship with psychoanalysis, and vice versa. This is because of fundamentally different perspectives on the origins of human behaviour. Neuroscience emphasises the almost mechanical, chemical functioning of the brain, while psychoanalysis stresses the more enigmatic phenomenon of the 'mind', as a lived experience of consciousness irreducible to quantitative data. Thus, neuroscientists hostile to psychoanalysis claim that although the technologies of measurement which have revolutionised neuroscience, such as MRI scans and other forms of bio-imaging, have demonstrated various functional states that do not require consciousness (for example, we can drive a car perfectly safely without being conscious of our every action), they have not provided *measurable* evidence of the existence of the dynamic unconscious described by Freudianism. On the other hand, those neuroscientists interested in some kind of *rapprochement* between these two perspectives – and this group seems to be growing – have pointed out the similarities between Freud's comments on memory, for example, and what has been discovered by neuroscience about 'implicit memory' (a form of memory which is not consciously recalled but is embedded in the performance of certain tasks). Despite the proposed convergence of the two disciplines, however, there are still many fundamental disagreements. Thus, insofar as neuroscience regards the brain as the locus of *material* interactions that can be positively measured and described, the sometimes vague notion of the unconscious can seem explanatorily useless, not to say downright obscurantist. Likewise, psychoanalysts who stress its clinical applications argue that the cold description of the brain as a kind of machine (albeit one with levels of consciousness) prevalent within neuroscience is of absolutely no use in therapeutic terms.

Political

Regarding the political objections to psychoanalysis, we have covered some of this ground already in the previous chapter. For such objections largely focus on a predominantly *normative* view of psychoanalysis, in which the claim is that psychoanalytic theory endorses a certain repressive social 'norm', and even imposes it through therapeutic 'discipline'. Such criticisms come from many political standpoints, but we can just mention three illustrative examples: feminists again, but also Marxists and Queer Theorists.

Thus, as we have already seen, feminists complain that psychoanalysis imposes an unjust, male-generated version of femininity upon women. Equally, Marxists, with their antipathy for the bourgeois ideology that disguises social contradictions under capitalism, argue that psychoanalysis is normative about bourgeois values, and therefore helps to perpetuate the injustices of capitalist exploitation. So, a Marxist might point out that the 'family romance' at the heart of orthodox psychoanalysis reflects a typically bourgeois family structure, the job of which is to maintain and perpetuate the existing 'relations of production' as well as certain ideals, such as the work ethic and social aspiration, etc.. Or they might argue that, in its emphasis on the individual, psychoanalysis reinforces the aggressive individualism that characterises the cultures of capitalism, and so on.

Equally, Queer Theorists (who generally advocate the social construction of gender roles) complain that psychoanalysis is normative about heterosexuality. At the level of theory then, psychoanalysis underlines the conservative assumption that (ideally monogamous) sexual relationships between men and women are the 'natural' status quo, whereas same-sex relations are always forms of 'perversion'. At the level of its clinical practice, psychoanalysis therefore potentially threatens the homosexual patient with increased, not reduced, anxiety. Or in a less essentialist mode, we might simply say that the heterosexual bias within psychoanalysis constrains the creative expression of a much more fluid and complicated sexuality that exceeds biological pigeon-holes like male and female, as well as gender pigeon-holes like masculine and feminine. For in either case, although 'unconscious homosexual urges' might be perfectly normal from a certain psychoanalytic perspective (as, for example, the residue of a partially unresolved Oedipal phase), such urges would still be viewed as something that needed to be 'worked through'. Indeed, 'conscious' and very deliberate homosexual behaviour – either as the reflection of a 'hard-wired' sexual preference, or as the expression of a performative mode of sexuality and identity – is always likely to clash with the heterosexual norm imposed by psychoanalysis (according to this line of criticism).

In each of these cases, it is the normative dimension of psychoanalysis that is being stressed, specifically that aspect which asserts that 'good' repression is the basis of mental health. Feminists, Marxists and Queer Theorists are simply pointing out that the moment one distinguishes a 'good' from a 'bad' form of repression, one is making a political decision which invariably draws on certain (perhaps we can still say 'unconscious') assumptions. These, in their turn, invariably favour one group over another. These are *political* criticisms of psychoanalysis both because they describe the plight of a group which might be considered a 'constituency', and because they are part of a wider attempt to push for changes that will address this plight. All three positions make polemical 'capital' out of the notion that psychoanalysis – as a body of ideas, a pervasive cultural influence, and a clinical practice which 'disciplines' those on the peripheries of so-called normality – can serve as a weapon in the armoury of today's patriarchal, capitalist, and 'hetero-normative' society. In other words, psychoanalysis lends itself to becoming a technology of control in the service of conservative forces.

Ethical

The ethical dangers of psychoanalysis are perhaps most obvious in the clinical setting. As Freud's 'seduction theory' demonstrates, therapy undoubtedly has the potential to introduce emotional turmoil not only into the lives of individuals undergoing analysis, but into the lives of their friends, their partners and their families. In common with religious clergy, psychoanalysts present themselves as morally resolute and dependable people to whom the care of spiritually and emotionally vulnerable individuals can be entrusted.

Indeed, the need for impeccable professional behaviour is arguably greater in the case of psychoanalytic therapy than in that of the priesthood, precisely because psychoanalysis operates by laying bare raw emotions and difficult memories. The analyst has an ethical obligation not to take advantage of sensitive phenomena which psychoanalysis itself both describes in theory and induces in the therapeutic situation. A prime example would be 'positive transference'. Because of the projection of intense feelings onto the person of the analyst, it is common for patients to go through a phase of believing themselves to be in love with their analyst (Freud, with a touch of narcissism, complained about this a lot). It is all-too easy to imagine how an unscrupulous analyst might use, or rather abuse, this situation.

But even if an analyst is far from being a manipulative sexual predator, there remains the corollary danger of 'counter-transference', in which the analysts themselves project their own unresolved feelings onto their patients. After all, analysts are also human beings with their own emotional and psychological dimensions. Occasionally, a situation may arise in which something an analysand says during analysis accidentally triggers a symbolic 'domino effect' for the analyst, encouraging them to invest their own emotions (perhaps even neuroses?) in the very person they are being paid to treat! Although followers of Klein have seen this as a positive tool in therapy, Freud felt this to be very precarious territory indeed. This is one of the reasons why Freudian therapists often go out of their way to cultivate a bearing not of warm intimacy, but of cold distance, in order to provide a neutral 'screen' for their patient's projections, and to fend off the dangers of both transference and counter-transference.

However, even if analysts are morally and emotionally self-disciplined, and even if they observe the most decorous behaviour imaginable, there is still the danger that in doing their very jobs to the best of their ability, they may be subjecting the analysand to a reductive form of violence. That is, it may be that precisely as *good* analysts, their talent lies in squashing the specificity of a complex individual into a relentless interpretative system, like mincemeat into a sausage machine. In fact, only bad analysts practice this clunky, mechanistic application of psychoanalytic theory, insensitively subsuming the patient's most intimate and painful confessions beneath utterly impersonal headings like the 'father-complex' or the 'depressive position', and so on. Yet perhaps this is a danger implicit in the very hermeneutic power of psychoanalysis? The French philosopher and trenchant critic of psychoanalysis, Gilles Deleuze, describes this ethical problem well:

> As soon as one begins analysis, one has the impression of talking. But one talks in vain; the entire psychoanalytic machine exists to suppress the conditions of a real expression. Whatever one says is taken into a sort of tourniquet, an interpretative machine; the patient will never be able to get to say what he really has to say.[3]

This is a strong criticism indeed, for it turns the apparently ethical basis of psychoanalysis, as an open and profoundly emotional exchange, into something closed and indifferent. Deleuze is suggesting that, despite appearances, psychoanalysis is not about communication at all: the analysand never really speaks, and the analyst never really hears. In point of fact, beneath the famous talking cure, there is a kind of sterile silence.

Arguments For Psychoanalysis

Having given ample room to some of the more significant personal, theoretical, political and ethical criticisms of psychoanalysis and of psychoanalysts, I would now like to balance the scales somewhat by qualifying these criticisms, and by making positive arguments for the value and importance of psychoanalysis today, addressing the same four areas as above.

Personal

The first and most obvious thing to say about the personal approach to criticisms of psychoanalysis is that it is an *ad hominem* mode of argument that is therefore necessarily reductive. To reduce psychoanalysis to the personality traits of its founder is to overindulge Freud's own paternal fantasies about being solely responsible for the genesis and subsequent institutional consolidation of psychoanalysis. I hope I have registered Freud's importance here, but no misguided 'cult of personality' should disguise the fact that Freud was synthesising the various intellectual

[3] Deleuze, Gilles. *Desert Islands and Others Texts: 1953-1974*, trans. Michael Taormina (Los Angeles: Semiotext(e), 2004), p. 274.

influences to which he was exposed, that his clinical development was nearly always in practical collaboration with others, and that, perhaps most importantly, the entire psychoanalytic movement has been greatly enriched and developed by many other minds since Freud. Besides, particularly in the realm of the history of ideas and of culture, isn't it deeply unsatisfactory to assess an original contribution on the basis of its creator's personal foibles? Would the Sistine chapel be any less beautiful if reliable historical evidence emerged proving that Michelangelo suffered from chronic flatulence? Or would Shakespeare's plays have to be abandoned if it emerged that the Bard was a womanising drunkard? When it does not connect personal failings to intellectual or artistic content, the personal approach always threatens to fall into this trap.

Regarding the personal attack on Freud's *scientific* credentials, it is worth staying within the criteria of the personal approach here by pointing out that such an attack would undoubtedly have been extremely distressing to Freud himself. He was, certainly in spirit, a scientist through and through. Far from glorifying the ineffable or celebrating the *mystery* of the human condition then, he was still substantially an Enlightenment thinker who believed in the capacity of reasoned inquiry to shed light on our deepest questions. Indeed, his first major project, in the days before psychoanalysis, was entitled *Project for a Scientific Psychology* (1895): it was an attempt to describe the workings of the mind in purely physiological terms, making psychology a natural science like biology or physics. It was the *scientific* as well as logical failure of this project that set him on the path towards psychoanalysis. And although he expresses a keen ambition to shore up the scientific rigour of psychoanalysis, this is tempered by some very honest assessments of its shortcomings in this regard. Indeed, in striking contrast to the megalomania sometimes imputed to Freud, his works are also littered with innumerable confessions of ignorance and even bafflement. He was not afraid to admit when psychoanalysis was throwing up more questions than answers. As a fledgling 'science', this was in fact usually the case: Freud was to some extent fumbling in the dark, literally making things up as he went along. And yes, he reached out for intellectual support to people like Jean Martin Charcot and Wilhelm Fliess. But isn't it a little uncharitable to see this as evidence of lack of scientific rigour? Instead, one ought to view it as the pioneering scientific spirit personified: Freud was making a very brave and very lonely foray into previously uncharted territory.

However, it bears repeating that the personal approach to criticisms of psychoanalysis is necessarily partial, and that Freud is far from being the beginning and end of psychoanalysis. Yet no other analyst has been subjected to the *ad hominem* form of critique as much as Freud, despite the numerous other analysts, from Alfred Adler to Donald Winnicot, from R. D. Laing to Julia Kristeva, who have taken psychoanalysis well beyond its

Freudian origins.

Theoretical

Let us tackle the theoretical broadsides against psychoanalysis's scientific credibility head-on. Here, in fact, contemporary science comes to our aid, because the rather Newtonian understanding of science that underpins many of these criticisms is, if not outdated, then increasingly supplementary to a very different understanding of science.

Since the revolutions in Quantum Theory and Chaos Theory in the latter half of the twentieth century, certainty just hasn't had the scientific currency it once enjoyed. Because of the increasingly acknowledged effects of complexity not only on ordered (yet always already disordered) systems, but also on the conduct of scientific observation itself, the data accruing from repeatable tests has become somewhat subservient to a more speculative approach to scientific problems. Cutting-edge science tends more and more to proceed by way of theoretical hypotheses that seem to have large descriptive scope in relation to observable phenomena, even if no concrete experiment can be designed to prove the hypothesis. Take 'Super-string Theory', which very clever people like Stephen Hawking take quite seriously. This theory posits not the point-like particles which we are used to imagining as pool balls bouncing off one another, but one-dimensional strings that are infinite, or link with themselves in loops, or curl into corkscrew shapes, all oscillating at various frequencies at the sub-atomic level and possibly traversing parallel universes! To the lay person, this all sounds very fanciful indeed. Moreover, no experiment exists that can definitively prove the reality of such tiny strings. However, 'Super-string Theory' has been popular among some scientists since the 1970s because it seems to describe all sorts of phenomena at the quantum level. Nonetheless, all that can be said with certainty is that some of the things that 'Super-string Theory' predicts do seem to happen, although this may yet be for reasons completely unrelated to tiny oscillating threads of matter.

This is not simply an example of a 'whacky' theory that enjoys widespread scientific credibility today (but which may, in time, look as crazy as Fliess's 'vital periodicity' does now). It also echoes Freud's own procedure in the formulation of his own cutting-edge 'science'. For Freud also found that the notion of the dynamic unconscious had a broad descriptive power which, despite falling short of hard proof, nonetheless lends a certain weight of probability in favour of its accuracy. Thus, the comparatively simple notion of the unconscious was able to explain extremely diverse phenomena of everyday life, from parapraxes to dreams, from neurotic symptoms to social psychology, and from sexual perversion to religious dogmatism. In a sense, Freud was applying the old scientific dictum of 'Occam's Razor', which says that out of a range of possible solutions to a problem or set of problems, the simplest is probably the best. Freud found that the unconscious was the simplest way to explain a vast spectrum of human behaviour, even to the extent of having a certain predictive value, and this fact in itself made its existence more likely.

In fact, by using himself as his own experimental guinea-pig in the early exploratory days of psychoanalysis, Freud was also, arguably, ahead of his time precisely as a scientist. For part of the same quantum revolution in science today is the rigorous acknowledgment that there is really no such thing as scientific neutrality or objectivity anyway, because the observer *does* always alter what s/he observes. This is the famous 'Heisenberg' or 'uncertainty principle' which has become a kind of shibboleth of quantum physics: it states that in measuring something, the very intervention of the act of measuring may distort the results. For example, to locate an electron, you have to bounce a photon off it, but the impact of the photon will alter the location you were searching for in the first place! You will measure, in part, the effect of the act of measurement itself! This does not mean that knowledge is impossible, but it does mean that it becomes unavoidably qualified: one has to acknowledge the effect of an unknowable variable on one's results. Now, clearly none of this applies very directly to Freud and psychoanalysis because such odd phenomena occur only at the quantum level. Yet it is important to register that all science is now less presumptuous about the objectivity of the scientist. Psychoanalysis could be said to have been ahead of its time in this very specific sense, because it always dramatised the problematic distinction between 'subject' and 'object'. Whereas the old Newtonian approach demanded the strictest separation between the 'subject' (the scientist) and the 'object' (the thing the scientist was observing), psychoanalysis makes a point of always acknowledging its 'object' (the human mind) as a 'subject' (again, a human mind). Moreover, in the emotional dynamics of the therapeutic setting, psychoanalysis carefully thematises the necessary exchange of mutual influence between 'subject' (this time as analyst) and 'object-subject' (the analysand), and one could argue that, on a very different level, this is what the quantum revolution has started belatedly to realise within scientific discourse.

Of course, this is not enough to get psychoanalysis 'off the hook' in terms of its theoretical and methodological rigour. The challenge that we have already noted coming from neuroscience is a real one: psychoanalysis undoubtedly struggles to meet the positivist demand, rightly still important in the harder sciences, for repeatable, measurable proof. In a context in which reality is increasingly measured by its capacity for visualisation (if we can represent it pictorially, it is real), whole warehouses of clinical case-notes attesting to the existence of the unconscious will not have the same persuasive power as a single MRI scan *showing* the unconscious at work.

Currently, we have no such image (and to look for one may already be to misunderstand the nature of the unconscious). In a sense, too, psychoanalysis faces a challenge on another front, from the massive advances in genetics and genetic engineering. For the extent to which human behaviour is shown to be pre-determined by genetic inheritance is also the extent to which the emphasis in psychoanalysis on environment, experience and memory is undermined. Furthermore, the extent to which genetic engineering, as an intervention into that 'pre-determination', might potentially 'manufacture' personality types is also the extent to which the *ad hoc* and piecemeal fine-tuning of the self in analysis may be rendered less necessary.

Yet these positivist scientific perspectives, which uphold a faith in their capacity exhaustively to explain everything about human behaviour, either by neurological patterns or by genetic predisposition (or both), miss a very fundamental part of the human *condition*. That extra, philosophical ingredient relates to the existential *experience* of consciousness that no MRI scan or genetic fingerprint can capture. The German philosopher, Martin Heidegger, argued that what is so different about human beings is that they are the only type of being for whom existence is an issue or a problem. We worry about why we are here and what the purpose of life is in a way which you wouldn't catch your average domestic cat wasting its energy on! And strangely enough, *seeing* an MRI scan of one's thought processes or having one's past explained or one's future mapped on the basis of genetic orientation has little or no salutary impact on this basic condition of philosophical anxiety. We do not feel 'better' for having ourselves explained to ourselves in this way. Indeed, information or knowledge seems to brush only very lightly against the surface of what it *feels* like to be conscious. Although neuroscience has made such tremendous advances in understanding the underlying processes of consciousness, then, it cannot unlock the existential conundrum of *being* conscious. One is reminded here of Jack Nicholson's great line in *As Good As It Gets* (1997), when, in a state of emotional pique he exclaims to his well-intentioned friend, 'I'm drowning here, and you're describing the water!'

Political

As already stated, the political objections to psychoanalysis almost always rest upon a normative reading of it. This reading, as we pointed out in the previous chapter, can be alleviated by an understanding of psychoanalysis that recognises its astonishing *descriptive* power. The extremely detailed and analytical attention that psychoanalysis has given to the very problems of patriarchy, bourgeois ideology and 'hetero-normativity' of which feminists, Marxists and Queer Theorists rightly complain (even if not from the same consciously politicised positions or using the same charged terminology), represents an invaluable theoretical resource for each of these interconnected political theories. Indeed, it is not simply that psychoanalysis provides tools in the 'kit-bag' of political activism and critique: it is also that psychoanalysis has within it a strong critical thread and an associated emancipatory potential.

Freud himself shed a great deal of light on the relationship between the super-ego and punitive power, and also between domination and the subject's masochistic willingness to surrender him or herself to that domination. Such interpretations of the psychology of power became all the more significant after the two great totalitarian follies of the twentieth century: Hitler's Nazism in Germany, and Stalin's totalitarian Communism in Soviet Russia. The respective pathologies of these two monolithic ideological systems (equally deserving of the clinical diagnosis of insanity) demanded interpretation, and psychoanalysis has proved equal to this task. Thus, studies like *The Authoritarian Personality* by numerous critical theorists from the Frankfurt School attempted, in the 1950s, to use psychoanalytic theory to explain the psychology behind fascistic personalities (like those of Hitler and Stalin), as well as the group psychology of violence behind the mass participation, by ordinary German citizens, in anti-Semitic atrocities during the period of the Third Reich.

Another critical theorist, Herbert Marcuse, proposed, during the same decade, a creative articulation between Freudianism and Marxism in his famous book, *Eros and Civilisation*. Here, Marcuse uses Freud's idea that society creates the energy it requires by repressing libido to talk about the renunciation of pleasure that the worker must undertake to be productive. Capitalism, claims Marcuse, imposes a surplus-repression on people in order to mobilise their productive forces. The particular form taken in this type of society by the reality principle, which Freud always thought of as a way of adapting to external constraints, is now the 'performance principle', whereby everything is measured for efficiency. For Marcuse, this is a very inhuman way of looking at social life. His proposed alternative, an 'aesthetic' model which emphasises play, sensuality and creativity, and thus a kind of eroticisation of labour (and everything else), was very influential during the so-called sexual revolution of the 1960s, when 'free love' was considered, naïvely perhaps, to be an alternative to the stoic moralising of a previous (war-time) generation. And of course, the feminist movement of the 1960s and 1970s in particular built on Marcuse's articulation of Freudianism and Marxism in order to address female identity, deploying psychoanalysis both critically (Simone de Beauvoir, Luce Irigaray) and creatively (Julia Kristeva, Juliet Mitchell, Judith Butler).

Political theory since the 1970s and 1980s has been more influenced by Lacanian theory than by Freudianism. Thus, Ernesto Laclau takes Lacan's idea of the constitutively 'unfinished' subject and uses it to construct a radical version of democracy that doesn't assume a unified subject as the primary unit of its 'raw material'. In general, Lacan's notion of the role of the 'Other' in establishing the self has been used, particularly in postcolonial theory, to examine the construction of identities, including national, religious and ethnic identities. In this way, it is possible to use psychoanalysis to shed light on why societies react in the ways they do to the increasingly unavoidable modern phenomena of immigration and asylum. How we treat our 'Others' reveals a great deal about how we think of ourselves. Another very important way in which Lacan in particular has influenced today's political theory is in his emphasis on desire and lack, and how these relate to contemporary pathologies. As we saw in chapter 8, Lacan suggests that in becoming subjects, we necessarily institute a lack at the core of our being, and that this in turn creates a desire that is incessant and can never be satisfied. Theorists of today's consumer society find this a useful description of the psychology of consumption, which is in many ways utterly irrational.

For example, given the choice between two identical white t-shirts, one at £5 in price, the other at £20, many brand-conscious consumers will buy the expensive one with the logo on it, even though they simultaneously know that there is no empirical difference in quality. Introducing the idea of unconscious desire helps to explain this phenomenon: logos cleverly condense sets of values, typically invoking a whole imagined lifestyle characterised by affluence, social success and fun, that consumers believe they are 'buying into' through their purchase of products marked by these logos. Rationally of course, we know this to be completely untrue. We all know that buying this or that t-shirt will not make us rich, happy and loved by everyone, yet *part* of us, our unconscious, does actually believe this myth to be true. So today's consumer culture is extremely adept at harnessing our unconscious desires and influencing our spending behaviour.

For political theorists with some allegiance to Marxism, this psychoanalytic dimension is important because it explains why, despite the predictions of Marxists, capitalism has not collapsed due to its own inherent contradictions. On the contrary, it is clear that capitalism is flourishing and, indeed, expanding rapidly in the form of globalisation. If the terrible exploitation that still seems to attend capitalism (just think of the gap between the developed and developing countries) is not *in itself* enough to lead everybody to rise up against it, this may be because capitalism has a particularly profound grasp of Lacanian desire. That is, consumer culture *simultaneously* plays on both our innate anxieties (making us feel undesirable and 'uncool') and on our narcissistic aspirations (to be cool, and therefore happy and complete), so that, in fact, it keeps us oscillating unhappily between feelings of inadequacy and ephemeral joy. As every shopaholic knows, the 'buzz' of the purchase soon wears off. Moreover, the consumer industries make sure that the goal posts are always moving, as it were, so that last season's clothes, although once cool, become the exact opposite as time passes and they threaten to suggest that you are not keeping up with changing trends.

Perhaps you might recognise aspects of yourself in this description? Nonetheless, this fact will probably not change your behaviour next time you are walking down the street. As we saw with neuroscience's explanation of consciousness, here again, knowledge is not sufficient on its own. This is one of the major messages of psychoanalysis, and it has proved useful to political theorists trying to understand today's consumerist society and the political apathy that some claim comes with it.

Ethical

If psychoanalysis has been extremely useful for political theory, it is also, I would suggest, ethically useful. Earlier, I used the analogy between priests and psychoanalysts to emphasise the ethical responsibility of the latter. Equally though, one could resort to the same analogy to point out that ethically negligent *individual* priests/analysts do not negate the value of the institutions which they represent (just as the existence of 'bad cops' hardly recommends the dissolution of the entire police force). What the existence of such individuals does indicate, however, is that the respective institutions ought to include very strict selection, training and monitoring procedures. Needless to say, the same thing applies to your local doctor.

Indeed, one of the primary purposes in the institutionalisation of psychoanalysis has been to establish standards of professional practice. For example, the American National Association for the Advancement of Psychoanalysis, or NAAP, which attempts to end the separatism of Freudians, Jungians, Adlerians and Lacanians by creating a single governing body, has rigorous codes of practice. These stipulate that analysts must maintain strict confidentiality, refrain from analysing friends or relatives, avoid engaging in sexual relationships with patients, and terminate analysis if a patient is not benefiting from it. The NAAP is sufficiently worried about such issues to have an ethics committee that oversees the implementation of these codes of practice, and this is far from unusual for psychoanalytic institutions. Although the factionalism characteristic of the various institutions of psychoanalysis has stemmed, very often, from disagreements about the right way to *train* analysts, the NAAP's guidelines nonetheless suggest a common awareness of the ethical sensitivity of the clinical setting. For whether they are Freudians, Jungians, Kleinians or Winnicotians, analysts must make very delicate decisions, particularly at the beginning of analysis. Is the patient's current suffering enough to justify the different kind of suffering that often comes with the revelation of difficult truths during analysis? Does the patient have a flexible enough ego to incorporate and build upon the often disorientating experiences gained through analysis? What is the support network around them like? Indeed, do they need psychiatric help, rather than psychoanalysis (or both)? Obviously, such questions bear particularly acutely on the future well-being of those individuals, by definition vulnerable, who turn to analysis. Part of the training to become an analyst is thus to fine-tune one's ethical sensitivity to the implications of one's decisions, actions and assumptions, and this is backed up, at the institutional level, by professional codes of conduct.

Moreover, it is a part of the very fabric of psychoanalysis to situate its own application of ethical behaviour within the social context in which it is conducted. After all, ethics reflect the values that govern what is deemed right and wrong by a given society or group. Because psychoanalysis must address wider social and ethical norms, it is not enough for the analyst, as an individual, to act in a way that s/he merely *feels* to be ethical. Rather, they must reflect on wider social values, and what assumptions these values include and perpetuate, and the extent to which their own practice reinscribes these assumptions. This is of clinical importance because neurotic symptoms, as we have seen, register a lack of fit between an individual and wider social norms. To have these norms simply reasserted in the clinical setting is of no therapeutic benefit to the patient.

But if psychoanalysis has to register the specific ethical composition of the environment in which it is conducted, the reverse is also true: the description of human nature offered by psychoanalysis has necessarily impacted on conceptions of ethics. This is because all ethical systems are based on a notion of human nature. The fact that Hobbes thought people were fundamentally cruel and brutish shaped his ethical thought, just as Rousseau's contrary conviction that people were fundamentally 'good' shaped his. Yet our understanding of human nature itself has changed with the advent of psychoanalysis. Indeed, one could also argue that, more than any other body of thought, psychoanalysis has described the structures and logics of *un*ethical behaviour. Notions like 'egoism', 'paranoia', and the 'death drive' go a long way towards explaining the psychology of immorality. The most basic tenets of ethical thought are impacted by these ideas. For example, within traditional ethical philosophy, freedom is a central concept, in so far as constraining the freedom of another is deemed unethical. Yet psychoanalysis emphasises the reciprocal and context-bound nature of all freedoms, so that the freedom of one individual is often a source of unfreedom for another. This is because psychoanalysis dirties its hands with the motivation behind the freedoms we actually desire, rather than some abstract Platonic ideal. For instance, in a flash of anger, I may want to be free to strangle my neighbour, but clearly this is unethical behaviour, not least because death is a fairly major constraint on freedom. In another sense, psychoanalysis is particularly good at explaining how we ourselves can be the primary agents of our own lack of freedom. For instance, I may experience my desire to strangle my neighbour as a real hindrance in my day-to-day encounters with him. Psychoanalysis might be able to tell me *why* I feel this disproportionate aggression, and even find a way to stop me feeling it.

To take another concept fundamental to ethics, and one that is bound up with freedom, the idea of choice (free or coerced) is also radically altered when viewed through a psychoanalytic lens. Without some notion of the unconscious, choice can be viewed as a conscious decision which draws on criteria for 'good' and 'bad' actions: an individual can *choose* whether to pull the trigger of the gun aimed at someone, or not. In many ways, the punitive dimension of the law assumes that individuals who make the wrong choice, thereby becoming criminals, should be punished for *consciously* doing something wrong. This assumes that the essence of ethical behaviour is about following rules. From such a simple perspective, apparently refusing to follow such rules is a deliberate refusal of the very principle of an ordered society. Yet, as soon as one introduces the notion of the unconscious, particularly in its inseparable relationship with aggression, one can no longer speak in such stark terms. Psychoanalysis suggests, then, that 'evil' may have a basis neither in individual delinquency nor in malevolent supernatural forces, but in 'instinctual urges', 'thanatos' or the 'return of the repressed', etc. Because not all the choices we make are conscious, we cannot simply treat decisions with 'bad' consequences as wilful disobedience.

But perhaps it is on the clinical level that psychoanalysis can best claim to be an ethical practice. After all, there is a lot of evidence (albeit not of indisputable scientific credibility) which suggests that, responsibly utilised, psychoanalysis can help individuals to gain self-understanding, confidence, and improved creativity.

Psychoanalysis Today

There are many arguments for and against psychoanalysis, and the controversy these debates generate looks set to continue to rage for a good time to come. For example, hasn't society itself changed almost beyond recognition since Freud's day? Haven't the prudish and hypocritical moral standards of the late Victorian era been swept away by a wave of liberalisation? How does the superego operate in a modern consumer society compared to its role within the patriarchal standards of old (assuming, that is, that they have really gone away)? Crucially then, if the times have changed, as they indubitably have, has psychoanalysis managed to change with them? This is too big a question to address here, but it is surely an important one to consider in evaluating psychoanalysis' contribution to our times. In fact, in reality, no simplistic 'for' or 'against' position is ever going to do justice to the complexity of what is a vast and diverse and, I would stress, *changing* movement. However, what is, I would venture, undeniable is that psychoanalysis cannot be simply discarded or discounted. Not even the harshest criticisms of psychoanalysis, whether centred on its sexual politics, scientific credibility, ethical implications, or indeed contemporary relevance, are in a position to dismiss it. This is because psychoanalysis remains one of the most important intellectual and cultural movements of the twentieth, and now twenty-first, centuries. It has had an incalculable influence over diverse fields, ranging from psychology to oil painting, philosophy to cinema, neuroscience to literature. In a very deep sense, psychoanalysis caused a kind of explosion deep within our conceptions of human nature itself, and the reverberations from this are still being felt today. Irrespective of its claim to be scientific, to articulate truths about the unconscious, to explain social phenomena, or to cure neurotic complaints, psychoanalysis *is* a major cultural influence that we all occupy.

Supplementary Bibliography

Works already cited in the text or footnotes do not appear here.

Bernard, Susan and Bruce Fink (eds.). *Reading Seminar XX: Lacan's Major Work on Love, Knowledge, and Feminine Sexuality* (New York: State University of New York Press, 2002).

Bruhle, Mari Jo. *Feminism and its Discontents: A Century of Struggle with Psychoanalysis* (London: Harvard University Press, 1998).

De Berg, Henk. *Freud's Theory and Its Use in Literary and Cultural Studies* (New York: Camden House, 2003).

DiCenso, James. *The Other Freud: Religion, Culture and Psychoanalysis* (London: Routledge, 1999).

Dufresne, Todd, *Killing Freud: Twentieth Century Culture and the End of Psychoanalysis* (London: Continuum, 2003).

Fink, Bruce. *Lacan to the Letter: Reading* Écrits *Closely* (London: University of Minnesota Press, 2004).

Freud, Sigmund. *Moses and Monotheism*, trans. Katherine Jones (London: Hogarth Press, 1939).

_____ . *Two Short Accounts of Psycho-Analysis*, trans. James Strachey (Harmondsworth: Penguin, 1962).

______ . *Case Histories,* trans. Alix and James Strachey (Harmondsworth: Penguin, 1979).

______ . *An Outline of Psycho-Analysis*, trans. James Stracey (London: W. W. Norton, 1989).

______ . *The Psychopathology of Everyday Life*, trans. Anthea Bell (London: Penguin Books, 2002).

Gay, Peter, *A Godless Jew: Freud, Atheism, and the Making of Psychoanalysis* (London: Yale University Press, 1987).

Gay, Peter (ed.). *The Freud Reader* (New York: W. W. Norton., 1995).

Hinshelwood, R., S. Robinson and O. Zarate. *Introducing Melanie Klein* (London: Icon Books, 1998).

Horowitz, Gad. *Repression: Basic and Surplus Repression in Psychoanalytic Theory: Freud, Reich and Marcuse* (Toronto: University of Toronto Press, 1977).

Hyde, Maggie and Michael McGuinness. *Introducing Jung* (London: Icon Books, 1999).

Irigaray, Luce. *This Sex Which is Not One* (Ithaca: Cornell University Press, 1985).

Jung, C. G. *The Archetypes and the Collective Unconscious* (London: Routledge, 1990).

_____ . *Psychological Types* (London: Routledge, 1999).

Klein, Melanie. *Our Adult World and its Roots in Infancy* (London: Tavistock, 1960).

_____ . *Contributions to Psycho-analysis, 1921-1945* (New York: McGraw

Hill, 1964).
_____. *The Psycho-analysis of Children* (London: Hogarth Press, 1975).
Kristeva, Julia. *Powers of Horror: An Essay on Abjection* (New York: Columbia University Press, 1982).
_____. *Black Sun: Depression and Melancholia* (New York: Columbia University Press, 1989).
Lacan, Jacques. *The Language of the Self*, trans. Anthony Wilden (New York: Dell Publishing, 1968).
_____. *Seminar XX, On Feminine Sexuality: the Limits of Love and Knowledge*, trans. Bruce Fink (New York: Norton, 1998).
_____. *The Four Fundamental Concepts of Psycho-analysis*, trans. Alan Sheridan (London: Vintage, 1998).
_____. *Écrits*, trans. Bruce Fink (London: Norton, 2006).
Lechte, John. *Julia Kristeva* (London: Routledge, 1990).
Mannoni, Octave. *Freud: The Theory of the Unconscious* (London: Pantheon Books, 1971).
Minsky, Rosalind. *Psychoanalysis and Culture* (Oxford: Polity Press, 1998).
Mitchell, Juliet. *Psychoanalysis and Feminism* (Harmondsworth: Penguin, 1974).
Nobus, Dany. *Jacques Lacan and the Freudian Practice of Psychoanalysis* (London: Routledge, 2000).
Robertson, R. and E. Timms. *Psychoanalysis in its Cultural Context* (Edinburgh: Edinburgh University Press, 1992).
Segal, Hanna. *Introduction to the Work of Melanie Klein* (London: Hogarth Press, 1973).
Segal, Julia. *Phantasy in Everyday Life* (London: Penguin, 1985).
Smith, Anne-Marie. *Julia Kristeva: Speaking the Unspeakable* (London: Pluto Press, 1998).
Thwaites, Tony. Reading Freud: Psychoanalysis as Cultural Theory (London: Sage, 2007).
Thurschwell, Pamela. *Sigmund Freud* (London: Routledge, 2000).
Ward, Ivan and Zarate, Oscar, *Introducing Psychoanalysis* (London: Icon Books, 2000).
Whitebook, Joel. *Perversion and Utopia: A Study in Psychoanalysis and Critical Theory* (Massachusetts: MIT Press, 1995).

Made in United States
Troutdale, OR
11/03/2026

56844905R00076